MW01096960

KIDNEY DISEASE DIET

This Book Includes:

Renal Diet CookBook and Kidney Disease Diet.

The First Complete Collection to Restore the Health of your Kidneys with a Healthy Diet and proper Lifestyle.

© Copyright 2019 - All rights reserved.

The content contained within this book may not be reproduced, duplicated or transmitted without direct written permission from the author or the publisher.

Under no circumstances will any blame or legal responsibility be held against the publisher, or author, for any damages, reparation, or monetary loss due to the information contained within this book. Either directly or indirectly.

Legal Notice:

This book is copyright protected. This book is only for personal use. You cannot amend, distribute, sell, use, quote or paraphrase any part, or the content within this book, without the consent of the author or publisher.

Disclaimer Notice:

Please note the information contained within this document is for educational and entertainment purposes only. All effort has been executed to present accurate, up to date, and reliable, complete information. No warranties of any kind are declared or implied. Readers acknowledge that the author is not engaging in the rendering of legal, financial, medical or professional advice. The content within this book has been derived from various sources. Please consult a licensed professional before attempting any techniques outlined in this book.

By reading this document, the reader agrees that under no circumstances is the author responsible for any losses, direct or indirect, which are incurred as a result of the use of information contained within this document, including, but not limited to, — errors, omissions, or inaccuracies.

Table of Contents

Kidney Disease Diet

Renal Diet Cookbook

Kidney Disease Diet

*Stop Kidney Disease
and Improve Kidney Function
with a Healthy Diet, a Correct Lifestyle
and the Latest Scientific Findings;
Includes the Renal Diet Cookbook*

Introduction

The kidneys, two bean-shaped organs located near the bottom of your rib cage, are rarely thought about by many Americans. Despite this, they are constantly helping us by filtering out waste and toxins, managing mineral content within our bodies, synthesizing vitamin D, and producing urine. Simply put, without our kidneys, we can't survive. These organs keep our blood clean and our bodies hydrated.

Sadly, more than thirty million Americans have chronic kidney disease. This disease, if left untreated, leads to kidney failure. This is why Dr. Robert Porter and Dr. Elizabeth Torres are bringing you the *Kidney Disease Diet* so that you can learn to treat and manage kidney disease, prevent kidney failure, and live a longer and healthier life.

You can learn all about the function of the kidneys, the effects of the disease, how inflammation impacts your body for better and worse, mineral overload, the importance of protein, and more from Dr. Porter. Along with this vital information, you can learn delicious and tasty recipes for the kidney disease diet from Dr. Torres. By utilizing the information and recipes from the pages of this book, you will find yourself on the path toward success.

Not only will you be able to treat your chronic kidney disease or CKD, but you will also be able to treat the conditions that commonly cause and worsen the disease, such as diabetes and high blood pressure. The sooner you make this change for the better, the more successful you will be in preserving your kidney function and health.

Chapter 1: The Power of the Human Kidney

Many people go through their lives, knowing very little about their kidneys. All they know are that they are two medium-sized organs (about the size of an orange) that are shaped similarly to a bean. You may even know that the kidneys are located on each side of your spine, directly below your rib cage. However, this is not enough information about these vital organs. After all, if you don't care for your kidneys, they can become diseased, leading to major health problems.

In this chapter, you will learn all about the importance of your kidneys, how they are constantly sustaining your body, and why you should protect them.

When your kidneys are healthy and capable of actively performing their duties, they will filter an average of four liquid ounces of blood every sixty seconds. While filtering this blood, the kidneys remove extra water which will be made into urine and any waste within the blood. After the water removes the water from the blood, it directs it to the bladder to become urine. This water is transported through the ureters, which are two thin tubes made out of muscle, located on each side of the bladder. This means that your kidneys, along with your bladder and ureters, are all a part of your urinary tract.

Many people mistakenly believe the kidneys act as sponges, which is far from the truth. The kidneys do not absorb and hold onto waste and harmful compounds. Instead, the kidneys filter out these toxins so that they can be completely removed from the body. They do this with a complex system that consists of millions of nephrons, which are microscopic filters. Nephrons are comprised of two components, which are the glomerulus and the tubule. In order to cleanse the blood, the glomerulus strains it of the larger molecules from fluid and waste. After these pass through the glomerulus, they head to the tubule. As the blood travels through the tubule component of the nephrons, smaller molecules of waste are collected. Not only that, but the tubule also collects any minerals found within the blood and then transfers them back into the bloodstream. But, how are these toxins removed from the kidneys and the body so that they don't stay stuck within your organs? When the kidneys filter water from your bloodstream, it combines the water with the filtered waste and toxins, therefore allowing them to be carried to the bladder before being expelled from the body.

Some of the waste that the kidneys remove from your blood is excess acid, which is produced in your blood in order to maintain healthy levels of minerals and water. This acid affects the levels of many minerals, such as potassium, sodium, calcium, and phosphorus. When these minerals are out of balance, your body will be unable to function properly. As these minerals are electrolytes, they affect the maintenance and control of your muscles, nerves, tissues, and balance.

Without the proper balance of these electrolytes, you can be in a rather dangerous situation.

Athletes are frequently aware of the importance of maintaining balanced electrolytes, as your body will naturally become depleted of these minerals as you sweat. This is the reason that sports drinks are popular. These drinks contain all the electrolytes the human body requires, allowing people to refuel on both water and minerals simultaneously. However, if you consume too many sports drinks or electrolytes in other forms, you will overload your blood and kidneys. It is important to contain a balance of electrolytes with neither too few or too many.

Along with filtering out water, maintaining electrolyte levels, and removing excess acid, your kidney provides other functions. This includes the production of red blood cells, blood pressure maintenance, hydration regulation, hormone production, vitamin D production for bone health.

Kidney Components

We've mentioned a few components of the kidneys, such as the glomerulus and tubule. However, it can easily become confusing and difficult to differentiate these various biological components. So, let's have a look at a list of all the kidney components for easy reference. If you ever get confused about all the biological terms simply refer to this list for clarity.

Nephrons:

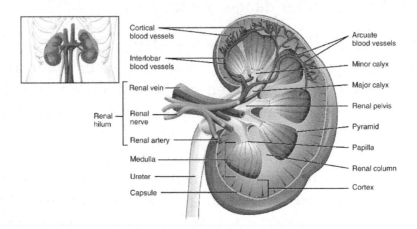

The most important aspect of the kidneys are the microscopic nephrons. Each of your kidneys contains around one million nephrons, whose job it is to filter blood, remove waste, and metabolize nutrients. Each of the nephrons contains its own set of internal structures.

Renal Corpuscle:

After blood is delivered to the nephrons, it is then processed by the renal corpuscle, which contains two additional elements. This is also known as the Malpighian body. The two additional elements of the renal corpuscle include the **glomerulus** and the **bowman capsule**.

The glomerulus, which is a cluster of capillary blood vessels, works to absorb protein from the blood as it travels through the renal corpuscle.

As the blood travels through the nephrons, the bowman capsule works to remove the excess water, known as capsular urine. The bowman capsule then transfers the capsular urine to the next portion of the kidneys, the renal tubules.

Renal Tubules:

The renal tubules are a connection of tubes that connect the bowman capsule to the collecting ducts. These tubules consist of multiple components, including the **proximal convoluted tubule**, the **loop of Henle**, and the **distal convoluted tubule**.

In the proximal convoluted tubule, water is absorbed while glucose and sodium are transferred back into the bloodstream.

The loop of Henle further absorbs sodium, potassium, and chloride in order to return them to your blood.

Lastly, the distal convoluted tubule absorbs more potassium and acid, while transferring more sodium into the blood.

By the time the renal tubules finish processing the water, or capsular urine, it is further diluted and full of urea. The urea is released into the urine as a byproduct of protein metabolism.

Renal Cortex:

The outer part of the kidney is known as the renal cortex, and it contains both the convoluted tubules and the glomerulus. Surrounding the outer edges of the renal cortex is a layer of fatty tissue, known as the renal capsule. The renal cortex works together with the capsule house in order to protect the kidneys and their inner structures.

Renal Medulla:

The smooth tissue located within the kidney is known as the renal medulla. The renal medulla works as a protective container for the renal pyramids and the loop of Henle.

Renal Pyramids:

These small structures within the kidneys contain and connection of tubules and nephrons. First, the tubules transfer water into the kidneys. Then, the water is directed away from the nephrons into the inner structures to transport and collect urine out of the kidneys.

Collection Ducts:

At the end of every nephron in the renal medulla is a collection duct. These ducts filter fluid as it leaves the nephrons and pushes it onward to its final destination within the kidneys, the renal pelvis.

Renal Pelvis:

In the innermost section of the kidneys is located the renal pelvis, which is a shaped like a funnel. The purpose of the renal pelvis is to create a pathway for urine to exit the kidney and head on its way to the bladder.

Calyces:

Within the renal pelvis is the calyces. These are small spaces that collect and hold water before it moves into the bladder. While in the calyces the water collects waste and further fluid, creating urine.

Hilum:

Within the opening inner edge of the kidney, where it curves inward creating its characteristic bean-like form, is the hilum. Within the hilum passes the renal pelvis, **renal artery**, and **renal vein**.

The job of the renal artery is to deliver oxygenated blood from the heart straight to the kidneys in order to be filtered.

The renal vein then delivers filtered blood directly from the kidneys and back to the heart.

Ureter:

Formed out of muscle tissue, the ureter is a tube whose purpose it is to push and deliver urine from the kidneys and into the bladder. After being delivered to the bladder, the urine is then collected and expelled from the body. While the kidneys process a lot of water during the course of a single day, only one or two quarts become urine. The remaining water is returned to your blood via the tubules to maintain hydration.

Overall, most peoples' kidneys will filter and process an average of one-hundred and fifty quarts of blood every day! As you can see, there are many components that make up your kidneys, and if any of them malfunction, it can lead to disastrous results. Any disease of the kidneys must be taken seriously.

The Kidneys and the Endocrine System

The human kidneys play an important role in the endocrine system, which is the production and control of hormones within the body. The kidneys are critical in the production of the hormone's renin, erythropoietin, and calcitriol. Not only that but they also synthesize prostaglandins, which affect various aspects of kidney function.

Along with the production and synthesis of hormones, the kidneys also participate in the degradation of hormones, including insulin and the parathyroid hormone.

Erythropoietin:

The erythropoietin hormone regulates the production of red blood cells. When this hormone is out of balance, a person's blood can either become dangerously thin or dangerously thick, which is potentially lethal if it is left without emergency medical intervention.

For adults, an average of ninety percent of their erythropoietin is formed and synthesized by the kidneys. The remaining ten percent is produced by the liver. While the liver plays a vital role in the production of erythropoietin during the fetal stages of growth, for adults, the liver is no longer able to compensate for lack of production in the kidneys. This means that if the kidneys fail to produce adequate levels of erythropoietin, the liver is unable to help maintain healthy levels of this hormone.

Most people who develop end-stage renal failure will experience anemia and a deficiency in erythropoietin. While doctors will sometimes administer blood thickeners to increase red blood cell production, it is not always effective.

Calcitriol:

Also known as 1,25-dihydroxy vitamin D3, calcitriol is a vital bioactive form of vitamin D3. This vitamin has important roles in the mineralization and health of bones, along with the regulation of phosphorus and calcium. However, there is a larger number of effects of calcitriol that are yet to be discovered, as it has been found to reside in a variety of cells.

Calcitriol is important for human health, as the body is unable to directly benefit from vitamin D absorbed from food or the sun. This "vitamin," is not a true vitamin but is actually instead a hormone. The vitamin D we absorbed from outside sources is delivered to the kidneys, where it is synthesized into the bioactive form of calcitriol. Once the calcitriol has been synthesized, it can then be used by the body to maintain homeostasis.

As kidney disease frequently causes a deficiency in calcitriol, many doctors will treat their patients with this hormone. In can be used to treat symptoms such:

- Hyperparathyroidism, an endocrine disorder characterized by excessive hormone production.

- Low blood calcium

- Osteomalacia, softening of the bone.

- Osteoporosis, degradation of the bones.

Calcitriol has a couple of other purposes, as well. First, it activates cell osteoblasts. This cell secretes the matrix needed for bone formation and also synthesizes collagen, needed for nearly all of the tissues, cartilage, and many other aspects of the body. Second, calcitriol helps to stimulate the small intestine, allowing it to then synthesize protein and absorb calcium.

Renin:

A part of the angiotensin-aldosterone system (RAAS), renin is an important component in kidney hormone health. After all, this system manages fluid balance, electrolyte balance, blood pressure, and systemic vascular resistance.

When there is a decrease in blood volume in the kidneys (causing low-blood pressure) as a result of insufficient blood flow your cells will begin to synthesis the renin protein and enzyme. The renin releases and alters several different enzymes and proteins, which have the end result of creating angiotensin II. This then causes the arteries to constrict, resulting in a rise of both diastolic and systolic blood pressure. Therefore, renin plays a vital role in raising low-blood pressure to a safe and manageable level.

Prostaglandins:

The prostaglandins are derived by the cellular metabolism of arachidonic acid to create a series of fatty acid hormone-like products. Unlike most hormones, prostaglandins are not created and then carried through the bloodstream to affect specific functions of the body. Instead, they are created by chemical reactions throughout the body wherever they are needed at the time. The purpose of these prostaglandins is to help the body heal from both illness and injury, making them a part of the inflammation response.

While chronic levels of high inflammation are damaging, as we will discuss later in this book, the inflammation response is still a vital part of the body. Without the inflammation response, we would be unable to heal or protect ourselves from harmful bacteria and viruses. They also manage blood clotting when we get a wound, so that we are less likely to bleed out. Not only that, but prostaglandins play an important role in the female reproductive system. This hormone controls the menstrual cycle, ovulation, and induction of labor.

But if prostaglandins are produced throughout the body as-needed what do they have to do with the kidneys? The kidneys are one of the many locations within your body that produce this hormone, and it plays an important role in kidney health. It turns out that the prostaglandins produced within the kidneys play an important role in overall kidney function. The process of the kidneys filtering waste, delivering minerals to the bloodstream, adding clean fluids back to the bloodstream, and transporting urine to the bladder is known as renal hemodynamics, and prostaglandins help manage this entire process. Without renal prostaglandins, the kidneys would be unable to function properly, creating dangerous side effects.

As you can see, the kidneys play several very important roles for overall health. This means that when something goes wrong with the kidneys, it can be quite dangerous, causing extreme symptoms. But what exactly could go wrong with your kidneys? First, when your kidneys are unable to function correctly, it can cause a buildup of fluid and waste within the body, along with excessive levels of minerals and electrolytes. This results in kidney disease, which can, later on, lead to high blood pressure, fluid retention, fatigue, and back pain.

There are many things that may cause the kidneys to become damaged or diseased. Some of the causes may be infections, various diseases, diabetes, or high blood pressure. The kidneys can also become damaged if there is a malfunction of the blood vessels leading to the kidneys, causing the organs to receive inadequate blood supply. As there is no one cause of kidney disease or damage, your doctor will have to diagnose not only your kidney disease itself but also the cause of the disease. It is vital that your doctor learns the initial cause; otherwise, they will be unable to properly treat it. For instance, if your kidneys are damaged due to the inadequate blood supply, your doctor will be unable to help if they are only treating you for diabetes. Thankfully, your doctor should be well-equipped to learn the cause of your disease if you have one.

Chapter 2: Kidneys Impacted by Disease

Kidney disease is infrequently thought about by people unless they have been diagnosed with it themselves. Yet, while many Americans go on their way, unaware an estimated thirty-seven million adults have been diagnosed with the condition. Not only that, but a person can feel fine and seem healthy and still be at a high risk of developing this disease if they don't take care of themselves, as millions of Americans are at risk. Thankfully, if a person is aware of the risk of kidney disease and the condition is detected early, it can help prevent the progression of the disease and potential kidney failure. Therefore, early diagnosis, treatment, and understanding of kidney disease and kidney health are vital.

People who are at the highest risk of developing chronic kidney disease are those with a family history of kidney failure, diabetes, and high blood pressure. The elderly, Latinx people, Native people, Pacific Islanders, and black people are also at an increased risk of developing kidney disease.

If your doctor suspects you might have kidney disease or that you are at an increased risk of developing kidney problems, they will check your blood pressure, urine albumin, and serum creatinine. Increased markers on these three tests usually result in a kidney disease diagnosis, but your doctor who is familiar with your individual case will be able to know for sure and officially diagnose you. Keep in mind that nobody but your doctor can diagnose you with kidney disease, even if your test results indicate you might have one.

If you are worried that you or someone you care about may have developed kidney disease then see your doctor right away, they will be able to run the necessary test to either confirm or deny whether you have the condition. Usually, both kidneys will be affected by the disease. As the kidneys become damaged, they will be unable to properly filter your blood, resulting in excess fluid and waste within your body. While there are often no symptoms present until the late stages of the disease, it is possible to experience side effects. We will cover these possible symptoms later on in this chapter.

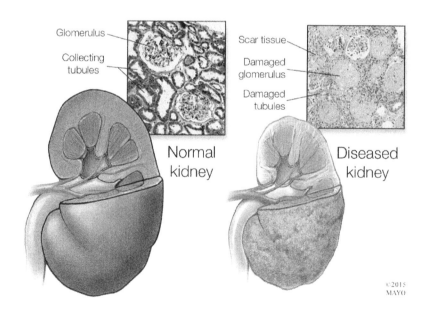

And, of course, you should be more careful of kidney disease if there is any history of it in your family. If you are concerned about an increased risk of developing the disease, ask your doctor about a plan to monitor your kidney health in the future to prevent any damage going unchecked.

Kidney Diseases and Illnesses

There are many different conditions that can cause kidney disease or overall poor kidney health. However, one of the most common and dangerous of these conditions is chronic kidney disease, also known as kidney failure. With this condition, a person's kidneys slowly lose their ability to function. If the person takes good care of their health, follows the treatment plans given to them by their doctors, and follows kidney health guidelines, they will hopefully be able to halt the progression of their kidney disease. On the other hand, if a person practices poor kidney health choices and goes without treatment, their kidneys will slowly deteriorate until they reach kidney failure.

When a person reaches kidney failure, the most severe stage of chronic kidney disease, the kidneys will be unable to function without medical intervention. In order to survive, people with kidney failure must either receive a kidney transplant or regular dialysis. Thankfully, healthy individuals are able to donate part of one of their kidneys or even a whole kidney to those in need without generally becoming sick themselves. This allows family members and friends to help their loved ones who are in dire need of a kidney transplant, and even kindhearted strangers who want to improve the world and do a good deed. If you are interested in donating part of your kidney, know that it is a common practice, and is one of the most common surgeries in the United States, making it a relatively safe procedure. If you are interested in donating a kidney or part of a kidney talk to your doctor, as they will know if your kidney is a good candidate for donation. They will also be able to discuss the safety and risks of your specific situation.

There are many conditions that can cause kidney diseases, such as inflammation of the kidneys, urinary tract obstructions, high blood pressure, and type I and type II diabetes. Kidney cancer is also extremely common, with it being the seventh most common type of cancer in the United States. There are also multiple types of kidney cancer, with renal cell carcinoma being the most common.

Kidney stones are extremely common and very painful, but generally, don't cause any damage. These stones are formed from minerals and acid found within the kidneys, usually making them a hard rock-like substance made of concentrated urine. Kidney stones usually pass on their own as long as you stay well hydrated. If you suspect you have a kidney stone and are unable to pass it on your own or worry that it might have caused rare damage contact your doctor and they can direct you further.

Another form of kidney illness is an infection of the kidneys. Usually, kidney infections are caused by bacteria that entered the body through the urethra, traveled through the bladder, and into the kidneys. Kidney infections can easily be treated, but if left untreated, they can cause permanent damage. Therefore, if you might have a kidney infection, seek medical attention immediately.

Along with chronic kidney disease, cancer, stones, and infections, there are some other kidney conditions, as well. If you suspect you have a kidney disorder that is not one of the ones mentioned above, your doctor will be able to discuss the possibilities with you and make a plan to figure out whether your kidneys have any problems.

Two-thirds of the cases of chronic kidney disease are caused by high blood pressure and diabetes. The reason for this is because diabetes, which occurs when your blood sugar is overly high, causes damage to your body. This results in damage to the kidneys and blood vessels, as well as the heart.

When a person has high blood pressure, known as hypertension, the blood in your veins pushes against the walls of the blood vessels. When left poorly controlled or uncontrolled, it cannot only result in heart attacks and stroke but also kidney disease. Along with high blood pressure causing kidney disease, kidney disease itself can also cause high blood pressure.

While two-thirds of the cases of chronic kidney disease may be caused by diabetes and high blood pressure, there are other causes as well. This includes repeated kidney infections, glomerulonephritis disorders, obstructions caused by kidney stones or tumors, polycystic kidney disease and other inherited diseases, Lupus, and malformations of a baby developing in a person's womb which results in pressure on the kidneys,

While there is no way to know for sure whether you have kidney disease without an official diagnosis from your doctor, there are some symptoms to keep an eye out for. It is important to understand our own bodies so that we can seek medical attention whenever there is cause for concern. By knowing and understanding these symptoms, you can inform your doctor of any concerns, which they can then keep an eye on to ensure you are in the best of health. After all, you will have the highest rate of success with treatment and lower risk of kidney failure if you get diagnosed and start treatment early.

Let's have a look at the most common symptoms:

1. **You feel fatigued and have trouble concentrating.**

   While this symptom is common with many illnesses, and simply in people who are overworked or not sleeping enough, it is important to note that it can be one of a myriad of symptoms that develop with kidney disease.

This is due to a buildup of toxins within the blood and possible anemia.

2. **Difficulty sleeping well.**

It can become difficult to sleep as toxins buildup in the blood rather than being removed from the body as they should. While sleep apnea is not a symptom of kidney disease, it is more common in people with this condition. This means that you could be suffering from poor sleep quality.

3. **Itchy and dry skin.**

There are many biological functions the kidneys play a role in. While the kidneys are largely known for their role of removing water and toxins from the blood, they also hydrate your body, maintain bone health, and produce red blood cells. If the kidneys are having difficulty maintaining the proper hydration in your body, then your skin can become dry, causing it to itch. This can also be a sign of worsening disease, as the advanced stage of the diseases can result in dry skin from an abundance of minerals and bone disease.

4. **There is blood in your urine.**

When your kidneys are functioning well, they are able to properly filter your blood, sending your blood back through your bloodstream and sending the urine to your bladder. However, when your kidneys become diseased, they have a more difficult time performing this task, and blood may escape into the urine. If you see blood in your urine contact your doctor, but don't jump to conclusions and assume you must have kidney disease. There are other common causes of blood in the urine, such as kidney infection and stones; your doctor will be able to discover what the cause of your blood is.

5. **You need to urinate more frequently.**

An increased need to urinate can have many different causes, such as urinary tract infections or an enlarged prostate. Although, sometimes this symptom is caused by chronic kidney disease, especially if this symptom is worse at night.

6. **Your urine is full of bubbles.**

When urine is full of bubbles, making it look foamy, it might require you to flush the toilet several times before the bubbles go away. This is an indication of protein in the urine, making it almost resemble thin egg whites. This is because the protein commonly found within urine, albumin, is the same type of protein in chicken eggs.

7. **Sore and swollen feet and ankles.**

When your kidneys aren't functioning properly, you can develop sodium retention, causing swelling in your tissues. This swelling will naturally pool in your feet and ankles, but might also pool in your hands at times. Keep in mind that swelling in the extremities is a symptom of many conditions and may be caused by something else altogether.

8. **Your eyes seem to always be puffy.**

Just as bubbly urine is a symptom of protein in the urine, excessive and prolonged puffiness around the eyes can be a symptom of the same. This is because the kidneys are failing to keep the protein in the body, where it is needed.

9. **Painful muscle cramps.**

Muscle cramps can have many causes, but one of the most common causes is electrolyte imbalance. If you have an electrolyte imbalance causing your muscle cramps it could simply be because you didn't properly rehydrate and fuel after sweating too much and developed an electrolyte deficiency or that you have kidney disease resulting in a buildup of electrolytes.

10. **You have little appetite.**

Again, this symptom can apply to many conditions and disorders. However, if you have been diagnosed with kidney disease and have a poor appetite, then your kidney disease may be the cause of this symptom. This is generally a result of increased toxin buildup in the body.

Side Effects of Chronic Kidney Disease

There are many side effects of chronic kidney disease, such as a buildup of toxins and minerals in the blood, fluid retention, anemia, and more. The disease, which is initially classified by kidney or renal insufficiency, may progress overtime into kidney failure. During the early stages of the disease, symptoms are uncommon, as while the renal tissue loses its ability to function, the remaining tissue will increase its function in order to maintain homeostasis. Yet, over time, the decreased function of the kidneys will lead to electrolyte imbalance and fluid retention, preventing the end goal of homeostasis.

In this portion, we will have a point-by-point look at the side effects caused by this disease. If you have been diagnosed with kidney disease, suspect you may have it or know someone with the condition, it is important to understand these effects.

Creatinine and Urea:

Creatinine is a product of waste formed when your muscles break down creatine. As it is your kidney's job to remove waste, including creatinine, an abnormal blood level of creatinine indicates irregular renal function.

Urea is primarily made in the liver, not the kidneys, but it plays an important part in kidney health. This is because the kidneys use urea to produce more concentrated urine. This is beneficial, as it allows the kidneys to redistribute cleaned fluid back into the body, only requiring waste to be expelled in a portion of liquid in the form of urine. This means that a person case maintains hydration and electrolyte levels more easily.

Concentrations of both urea and creatinine are indications of a renal malfunction, which is why a doctor will usually run a blood test as the first measure when checking for kidney disease. This test is known as the glomerular filtration rate (GFR) test. Diminished GFR indicates a problem. Initially, the concentration of urea and creatinine will be limited, but it will increase as the disease worsens.

Water and Sodium:

Initially, despite a decreased glomerular filtration rate (GFR), your body's water and sodium levels will maintain balanced. This is due to a normal thirst response and increased sodium excretion in the urine. This allows the blood to maintain the correct sodium balance while also staying hydrated. Unless a person overly restricts or exceed the recommended dietary intake of water and sodium, their hydration and sodium levels should appear normal.

Potassium:

The distal nephron, a portion of the kidney tubule, maintains secretion of potassium. Because of this, blood potassium levels typically maintain normalcy until a person develops kidney failure. Although, their potassium levels might be unnaturally elevated if a person is consuming more than their daily recommendation of potassium in their diet. Potassium may also be raised in patients with kidney disease if they take the following drugs:

- NSAIDs

- Beta-blockers

- Potassium-sparing diuretics

- Tacrolimus

- Cyclosporine

- Pentamidine

- Trimethoprim

- Angiotensin II receptor blockers.

Calcium, Phosphate, Vitamin D, and Parathyroid Hormone

A person may experience abnormalities in their parathyroid hormone, calcium, phosphate, and vitamin D levels with kidney disease. There are multiple potential causes of this, but a problem with one of these four components can trigger a cascade effect with the other three as they work in conjunction with one another.

Before changes in your phosphate, calcium, and vitamin D can be discovered through blood tests; your doctor may be able to detect an increase in the parathyroid hormone, known as hyperparathyroidism. Therefore, if you have kidney disease, it is important to closely monitor the parathyroid hormone, otherwise known as PTH. If your doctor can detect an excess of PTH, it can be treated before the abnormalities in your calcium, phosphate, or vitamin D become excessive.

Renal Osteodystrophy:

A bone disease caused when the kidneys are unable to maintain healthy phosphorus and calcium in the bloodstream; renal osteodystrophy is a disease commonly affecting people with kidney disease or who are on dialysis. This disease causes a high bone turnover rate, meaning that the body is forming and reabsorbing bones at an excelled rate, resulting in weakened bones and low bone mass. On the other hand, it may instead cause low bone turnover rate in some people, which is just as damaging as an increased bone turnover rate. Either way, your bones are damaged and weakened.

Bicarbonate and pH:

Metabolic acidosis is caused by a reduction of bicarbonate in the bloodstream, which causes an increase in acid due to a pH imbalance. Moderate metabolic acidosis is classified as a blood bicarbonate level of fifteen to twenty mmol/L. Your doctor can check for this side effect of kidney disease with a quick blood test. It is important to watch for, as metabolic acidosis can cause bone loss, muscle wasting, and an acceleration in the progression of chronic kidney disease.

Anemia:

Not everyone with chronic kidney disease will experience anemia, as it is usually not present until moderate to advanced stages. Due to a reduction in kidney function, a person usually becomes deficient in erythropoietin, which is the hormone produced in the kidneys to create red blood cells. However, a person may also develop anemia due to deficiencies in iron, vitamin B12, and folate.

Chronic Kidney Disease Diagnosis

Doctors usually first suspect chronic kidney disease when their patients exhibit an increase in their blood creatinine levels. They will then seek to discover whether the kidney failure is acute, chronic, or acute superimposed on chronic. This may seem confusing, but these three terms have very simple descriptions:

1. Acute: a condition experienced for a short period of time, but often to an intense degree.

2. Chronic: a condition that persists for a long period of time or persistently.

3. Acute superimposed on chronic: an acute disease that worsens renal function in a patient with chronic kidney disease.

Along with uncovering the duration of kidney failure, your doctor will search for the cause, as there are many potential causes. Sometimes, it is not easy to discover the duration of renal failure, and it might be easier to first discover the cause and then determine the duration from there.

Your doctor will test your urine, known as a urinalysis. The purpose of this is to get the details on your urinary sediment, phosphate, creatinine, calcium, urea nitrogen, and electrolytes. They will also run a complete blood count, which is important as many people with kidney disease will experience reduced red blood cell production. Sometimes, to determine the cause of your disease, a doctor will run specific serologic tests in order to search for certain antibodies. The easiest way to differentiate chronic kidney disease from an acute kidney injury is with a medical history of abnormal urinalysis or elevated creatinine.

A doctor may request an ultrasound to rule out acute kidney injury and to search for a urinary tract obstruction. While there are a few exceptions, most people with chronic kidney disease have shrunken kidneys that exhibit a thinned and hyperechoic cortex (the outer part of the kidney, between the renal capsule and the renal medulla).

It becomes increasingly difficult to make a precise diagnosis when the renal function declines to values close to end-stage renal disease. In this case, the definitive diagnostic measure is a kidney biopsy. Yet, a doctor might not be able to perform a kidney biopsy when an ultrasound indicates the kidneys are small with excessive fibrous tissue. In this case, the risks of the procedure will outweigh the benefits. Your doctor will be able to examine the ultrasound to determine whether or not a renal biopsy is needed, and if the benefits outweigh the risk or not.

There are five stages of chronic kidney disease, which doctors use to classify how damaged the kidneys have become, mark the progression of the disease, and indicate the severity of the side effects. A doctor will use the glomerular filtration rate (GFR) test in order to classify which stage a person is in.

- **Stage One**

- A person has normal GFR results ($\geq$ 90 mL/min/1.73 m2) along with either persistent excessive albumin protein in the urine, structural kidney disease, or hereditary kidney disease. Kidney damage may also be viewable through an ultrasound, CT scan, X-ray with contrast, and an MRI.

- **Stage Two**

- GFR results 60 to 89 mL/min/1.73 m2. At this point, the person is unlikely to be experiencing symptoms from the disease. Therefore, if the disease is discovered this early, it is often only due to the treatment of another disease, such as diabetes or high blood pressure.

- **Stage Three A.**

- GFR results 45 to 59 mL/min/1.73 m2. A person may start to experience symptoms during stage three (either type A. or B.). These may include fatigue, lower back pain, shortness of breath, swelling, fluid retention, urination changes, muscle cramps, restless legs, or trouble sleeping. These symptoms are the same in both types of stage three.

- **Stage Three B.**

- GFR results 30 to 44 mL/min/1.73 m2

- **Stage Four**

- GFR results 15 to 29 mL/min/1.73 m2. Along with the symptoms in stage three, a person may experience additional symptoms in stage four. These symptoms can include nausea, vomiting, loss of appetite, taste changes, bad breath, difficulty concentrating, and nerve problems such as numbness and tingling.

- **Stage Five**

- GFR results <15 mL/min/1.73 m2. Along with the symptoms of the previous stages, a person in stage five (kidney failure) may experience itching, skin color changes, puffy eyes, and little to no urination.

Once your doctor knows the cause of your kidney disease, the duration, and stage of kidney disease, they will be able to devise an individual treatment plan. While kidney disease can be scary if you follow the treatment plan and make beneficial lifestyle and diet changes, you can stop the progression of the disease and improve your prognosis in many cases. With a little knowledge, you no longer have to fear.

Chapter 3: Inflammation and Its Effects

When your tissues are damaged, your cells become inflamed. This is a natural and beneficial defense mechanism that allows the body to protect itself from injury and infection. The purpose of this inflammation is to remove damaged tissue so that the body can replace it with healthy tissue while also isolating and eliminate dangerous elements so that the body can heal itself. The inflammation response consists of a boost in the permeability of the blood vessels; altered blood flow; and relocation of fluid, white blood cells, and proteins to the location of the damage. If this inflammation only lasts for a few days or a week, it is known as acute (short-term inflammation), but if it lasts longer, it is known as chronic inflammation.

Acute inflammation is often beneficial and needed, although it can cause difficult and uncomfortable side effects. These side effects can vary depending on the extent of the inflammation, but it often causes pain, swelling, and itching. For instance, the swelling you develop after spraining a muscle and the itchiness from a bug bite or hives are both due to acute inflammation. Thankfully, this discomfort is often temporary and will dissipate as the inflammation response reduces.

However, while inflammation is generally beneficial and necessary, it can also cause harm to the body.

When the inflammation response becomes defective or excessive, it can cause damage to the tissue, pain, swelling, and other chronic side effects. At times, an inappropriate immune response can cause hypersensitivity and severe allergic reactions. For instance, hay fever and dangerous anaphylactic shock reactions are both due to an excessive and inappropriate immune response. Anaphylaxis is when a person experiences a severe allergic reaction to specific substances, for instance, peanuts or shellfish. This anaphylactic reaction can cause the throat to swell and is frequently lethal if left untreated. Excessive inflammation is also common in people with autoimmune illnesses, in which the inflammation response is triggered against the body's own healthy cells rather than dangerous foreign substances.

There are many different conditions and triggers that can instigate the inflammation response. This includes chemicals, microorganisms, physical agents, tissue death, and inappropriate immunological reactions. A couple of the most common instigators of the inflammation response are bacteria and viruses.

When bacteria enter the body, it releases substances known as endotoxins, which the body fights against with inflammation. Viruses damage and destroy cells upon entering the body, which causes inflammation to occur in order to isolate the damage, remove the damaged cells, and heal the location. Physical trauma, such as wounds and burns, cause tissue damage, inducing the inflammation response in order to prevent bacteria from entering the wounded tissue and to help health and replace the damaged cells. When tissue dies from lack of nutrients and oxygen, which can occur when blood flow is restricted from an area, inflammation again occurs.

There are multiple signs of inflammation. The four characteristic signs include swelling, heat, redness, and pain.

1. Swelling is also known as edema and is primarily a result of fluid accumulation outside of the blood vessel network.

2. Heat is caused by an increase in blood flow to a localized area. This heat is only caused on the surface of the body, such as on the skin. Although the chemical mediators of inflammation can also result in a rise in body temperature, triggering a fever.

3. Injuries and wounds will frequently become red, which is the result of an enlargement of the small blood vessels in the area.

4. The pain frequently associated with the inflammation response is caused by multiple factors. First, it is often caused by the distortion of your tissues resulting from the swelling in the area. Although, it is also caused by the chemical mediators of inflammation, such as prostaglandins, serotonin, and bradykinin.

The Acute Inflammation Process

There are many aspects that are involved in the inflammation response. It is important to understand this process if you want to utilize inflammation for healing without allowing it to cause damage itself. Inflammation is a powerful tool against disease, injury, and infection. But it is important to not allow it to become a double-edged sword, causing more harm than good. In this portion, we will examine the details of how the inflammation response works, allowing you to harness it to its full effect without unnecessary damage.

Vascular Alteration:

When your tissue is damaged the small blood vessels in the area momentarily constrict. This process is known as vasoconstriction. This is a fleeting and temporary constriction, which is believed to be of only slight importance to the overall inflammation effect. After the vasoconstriction, the blood vessels then enlarge, known as vasodilation. The dilation of the blood vessels increases blood flow to the area, allowing for better healing. This vasodilation can last for as few as fifteen minutes or up to several hours.

Usually, the walls of the blood vessels only allow sodium and water to easily pass through, to maintain hydration. Although, during this process they become increasingly permeable, allowing exudate, a protein-rich fluid, to easily pass through the walls of the blood vessels and into the damaged tissue. The exudate fluid contains various elements, such as clotting factors to prevent blood loss and the spread of infection, as well as antibodies, to destroy any possible invading microorganisms.

As the exudate exits the blood vessels, the flow of blood becomes more sluggish as it begins to clot in the area. White blood cells begin to fall away from the center of the blood vessels and begin to collect against the inner wall of the vessels.

Cellular Adaption:

Largely recognized as the most important factor of the inflammatory response is the collection of white blood cells at the location of the injury. The most prevalent of these white blood cells are the phagocytes, whose job it is to ingest foreign particles and bacteria while removing cellular debris from the injury site. The most common phagocytes white blood cells used in acute inflammation cases are neutrophils, which contain granules of proteins and enzymes that can destroy cells. If there is only slight damage, these neutrophils can be obtained from the blood vessels. Although, if there is extensive damage to the bone marrow, where these cells are produced, will release an increased supply of neutrophils.

The neutrophils exit through the wall of the blood vessels and then move toward the area of damaged tissue in order to complete their task. This movement through the blood vessels and tissue is possible due to a chemical substance, known as chemotactic factors, that release from the area of tissue damage.

This substance creates a concentration gradient, allowing the neutrophils to travel to their destination. This process is known as chemotaxis.

Shortly after the injury, a large number of neutrophils reach the site of injury or infection. Within an average of twenty-four hours after the neutrophils arrive another type of white blood cell enters the picture. This type of white blood cell is known as monocytes, which eventually grow into macrophages. These macrophages usually only become prevalent at the location after days or weeks of injury or infection, and they are a sign of chronic inflammation rather than acute.

Inflammation Chemical Mediators:

While injury or infection is the initiating factors of the inflammatory response, it is various chemical reactions and factors that stimulate the cellular and vascular reactions. These chemicals originate largely from the white blood cells, blood plasma, mast cells, platelets, endothelial cells, and damaged tissue cells.

One of the most well-known chemical mediators in this process are the histamines. These histamines trigger the enlargement of the blood vessels and increased the permeability of the vessels. The histamines are immediately released upon injury or infection from their stored location within mast cells and basophil white blood cells. This process is further achieved by the release of lysosomal compounds, which are released from the neutrophils white blood cells.

Prostaglandins, which are a group of fatty acids produced by various cells, play an important role in the inflammatory response. There are different types of prostaglandins, and each type has its own role. One type of these fatty acids manages platelets by forming them into clusters, activating the clotting process. Other prostaglandins affect other substances that are a part of the inflammatory response, allowing these substances to better promote vascular permeability. The pain and fever caused by inflammation are frequently associated with the release of prostaglandins. Anti-inflammatory medicines, such as aspirin, are effective in reducing pain and fever as they restrain the enzymes that are necessary for the synthesis of prostaglandins.

Blood plasma contains four interconnected systems of proteins that activate certain inflammation mediators. These are coagulation factors, kinins, fibrinolytic system, and the complement system. Let's look at a quick overview of these four aspects:

1. **Coagulation Factors**

2. The coagulation system transforms the plasma protein fibrinogen into fibrin. This is a major aspect of the fluid exudate, which allows for coagulation of the blood.

3. **Kinins**

4. The system of kinins is activated by the coagulation factors, which then produces substances to boost vascular permeability.

There are various types of kinins, and bradykinin is the most important. This type of kinin is the cause for much of the itchiness and pain experienced due to the inflammation response.

5. **Fibrinolytic System**

6. The fibrinolytic system helps the inflammation response by forming the enzyme plasmin. This enzyme's job is to break down the protein fibrin to create products to affect the permeability of the blood vessels.

7. **Complement System**

8. The activated proteins from the complement system help to move neutrophils white blood cells to their needed detestation, stimulate the mast cells to release histamines, and aid in vascular permeability. These proteins also stick to harmful bacteria, making it easier for the phagocyte cells to consume the bacteria, thus preventing them from harming your cells.

Following Acute Inflammation

After the acute inflammation response is triggered, there are multiple possible outcomes. These outcomes include the possibility of either repair and healing, suppuration, or chronic inflammation. Which of these three outcomes you experience depend on the tissue damaged, how much tissue destruction took place, and the cause of the injury. We will now examine the three possible outcomes, as they will affect whether you make a full recovery or begin to experience chronic side effects.

Repair and Healing:

During the healing process, damaged cells that can reproduce begin to regenerate. This ability to regenerate and reproduce will vary depending on the specific type of cell damaged. Epithelial cells are those which are frequently found on the surface of your body, such as on your skin and organs, and they are able to easily regenerate. On the other hand, the cells making up your liver do not easily regenerate, yet they can be stimulated to regenerate once the damage has occurred.

While there are many types of cells that can regenerate, for this regeneration to be achieved, it is vital that the structure of the tissue is easy to reconstruct. For instance, it is easy for your cells to regenerate simple wounds on the surface of your skin. It is more difficult for the cells to regenerate damage to complex structures, such as glands and organs.

Sometimes, if your cells are unable to properly regenerate the cells of an organ, it can lead to disease. For instance, this is the cause of liver cirrhosis and kidney failure. Since your cells are unable to heal your kidneys from the chronic disease, the damage to the cells increases while you advance through the stages of the disease, eventually leading to kidney failure.

When cellular damage is unable to be fully and successfully regenerated due to excessive damage, it results in the creation of fibrous scar tissue. During the repair process, endothelial cells cause the production of new blood vessels and cells known as fibroblasts, which grow to create a framework of connective tissue. This delicate tissue filled with blood vessels is known as granulation tissue. As time goes on and the cells continue the repair process, the new blood vessels create a network of blood circulation in the damaged area, along with fibroblasts building up increased collagen to help strengthen the weak tissue. Over time, the densely packed collagen creates scar tissue. This scar tissue usually of a lesser volume than the original tissue that it replaces, resulting in an organ that is distorted and contracted.

Suppuration:

When the body has difficulty eliminating the cause of inflammation, it will produce pus, in a process known as suppression. This pus is a thick liquid consisting largely of dying or dead bacteria and neutrophils white blood cells, along with cellular debris and fluid that has leaked from your blood vessels. The most common cause of suppuration is an infection from bacteria such as *streptococcus* and *staphylococcus*.

You may be familiar with these two bacteria, even if you do not know them by name. The first of these two bacteria, *streptococcus,* is the highly contagious bacteria responsible for strep throat. The second, staphylococcus, is a group of bacteria that cause dangerous staph infections. Both streptococcus and staphylococcus are known as pyogenic bacteria, meaning they are specific bacteria known to result in the production of pus.

Pus can be white or tinged with yellow, green, or pink. As it begins to collect in your tissue, it will become surrounded by a membrane, resulting in the formation of an abscess. This collection of pus, the abscess, is incredibly difficult to treat as it is inaccessible to both natural antibodies and antibiotics. In these cases, it may be necessary to receive a simple surgical procedure to lance the abscess and drain it of the pus. Other types of abscesses, known as boils, may burst and drain of pus on their own. Either way, once the pus has been drained the cavity of the abscess will collapse, allowing the tissue to repair and replace itself in the healing process.

Chronic Inflammation:

If the initiating cause of inflammation is unable to be eliminated, or if there is an obstruction to the healing process, then the acute inflammation may become chronic. Repeated instances of acute inflammation may also result in chronic inflammation. For instance, if a person experiences frequent kidney infection, the acute inflammation from the healing of the infection may become chronic, leading to chronic kidney disease. The exact duration, extent, and effects of this chronic inflammation will depend on the exact cause and a person's individual ability to repair the damage.

While acute inflammation is often a result of acute inflammation, this is not always the case. There are instances in which chronic inflammation is independent of acute inflammation, such as when a disease is present. For instance, chronic kidney disease, lupus, rheumatoid arthritis, tuberculosis, and lunch disease all may cause chronic inflammation without first causing acute inflammation.

When a person experiences an autoimmune reaction, they will develop chronic inflammation as a normal result of the immune system mistakenly attacking the body's own healthy cells. These autoimmune reactions result in the development of chronic inflammatory diseases, such as lupus.

The telltale sign of chronic inflammation is the occurrence of plasma cells, lymphocytes, and macrophages as the tissue site. These cells arrive from the circulatory system due to the release of chemotactic factors. While there are multiple types of cells released due to chronic inflammation, the hallmark of long-term inflammation is the increased presence of macrophages. These cells are usually beneficial, but when they occur in an excessive number during chronic inflammation, they contribute to increased tissue damage and impairment of the consequent function.

One type of chronic inflammation is especially damaging and disastrous, which is granulomatous inflammation. With this form of inflammation, modified macrophages, cells created small clusters, known as epithelioid cells. These often become surrounded by lymphocytes, a type of white blood cell, and may contain giant cells. This cluster of cells is known as a granulomas tissue. Some examples of when this granulomas tissue form is in the cases of tuberculosis, rheumatoid arthritis, syphilis, and fungal infections.

Inflammation of the Kidneys

There are various conditions that can cause inflammation in the kidneys. This is known as nephritis, which is a term that originates from Greek. The first part of nephritis is derived from "nephro," meaning "of the kidney." The second half of the word, "itis," means "inflammation." There are many different potential causes of nephritis, such as toxins, infections, and autoimmune disorders. Some of these conditions include lupus nephritis, glomerulonephritis, interstitial nephritis, pyelonephritis, and yes, chronic kidney disease.

While there are several potential causes for chronic inflammation of the kidneys, in this portion, we will focus on inflammation as a result or accompanying chronic kidney disease.

Chronic inflammation of the kidneys can occur in people with chronic kidney disease, which can then lead to dangerous cardiovascular disease and increased mortality risk. A 2015 study from Weill Cornell College of Medicine in New York, found that chronic inflammation is common in people with chronic kidney disease, and should be considered a comorbid condition. They surmised that people with chronic kidney disease should be watched for chronic inflammation, especially if the patient is on dialysis. Thankfully, with proper treatment, this can be greatly reduced and managed.

Some of the causes of nephritis in people with chronic kidney disease include the following:

- Poor nutrition due to poor diet or appetite

- Anemia

- Kidney transplant failure

- Extra waste in the blood, known as uremia

- Vascular infection at the access point for dialysis

- Poor dental health or gum disease

- Foot ulcers

- Toxins and pollutants

- Obesity; especially focused around the abdomen

- Lingering infections

- Insomnia or poor sleep quality

- Absence of exercise

A common connection between chronic kidney disease and chronic inflammation is malnutrition or poor nutrition. After all, it is common for people with kidney disease to develop symptoms that lead to difficulty eating, especially if they are in the late or end stages of the disease or are on dialysis. When a person develops a poor appetite, nausea, or vomiting, it results in a lack of poor nutrition, decreased protein intake, and a decline in calorie intake. As this decrease in nutrition continues overtime, the patient can develop protein-energy malnutrition, sometimes referred to as PEM. When a person develops this condition, their muscles are broken down in order to provide fuel for the vital functions of the body, as it is not receiving enough protein through dietary intake. This, in turn, results in weight loss and muscle wasting. To determine the severity of protein-energy malnutrition a doctor can

To prevent and treat chronic inflammation with chronic kidney disease, you first need to begin with a healthy, balanced, and kidney-friendly diet. This includes a focus on protein and adequate calorie intake to prevent malnutrition, along with antioxidant-rich foods, to overcome the inflammation. This diet will also regulate the amount of sodium, potassium, and phosphorus you consume to prevent an overload of these vitamins in your system.

Along with a healthy kidney disease diet, a doctor may prescribe medicines to counteract and treat chronic inflammation. Yes, over-the-counter medicines, such as NSAIDs, can treat inflammation. However, you should not treat your inflammation with any medication without first discussing it with your doctor. After all, NSAIDs can reduce inflammation, but they also have their own side effects and are usually not recommended for people with kidney disease unless specifically recommended by their doctor. There are different types of NSAIDs on the market, but some of the more common options are Ibuprofen, Aspirin, and Aleve. Always discuss any medications, even those that are sold over-the-counter, with your doctor before you begin taking them. Medications that are generally safe for healthy people can cause negative side effects in those with kidney disease and other illnesses. For instance, people with decreased kidney function may develop acute kidney failure due to NSAIDs. Only your doctor and pharmacist can determine if these medicines are safe and appropriate for your individual case.

Chapter 4: Renal Metabolic Acidosis

A common complication of chronic kidney disease is metabolic acidosis. Not only does this condition frequently occur because of kidney disease, but evidence now shows that it can also be a contributing factor to the worsening progression of the disease. Therefore, it is vital that any acidosis is treated and managed as soon as possible. Metabolic acidosis develops when a person's body produces excessive natural acid or when the kidneys fail to function properly and remove enough acid from the body.

Even if a person does not have renal metabolic acidosis, simply having an excessive dietary acid load can worsen kidney health. Thankfully, studies have shown that treating metabolic acidosis with acid-neutralizing agents can be effective, treating both the acidosis and slowing the progression of the disease.

There are different types of metabolic acidosis. For instance, there is diabetic acidosis caused by an excessive buildup of ketone bodies, hyperchloremic acidosis from excessive sodium buildup, lactic acidosis from a buildup of lactic acid, and renal metabolic acidosis. In general, the only one that people with chronic kidney disease have to worry about is renal acidosis. Of course, if the person has other condition as well, such as diabetes, then they will also be predisposed to diabetic acidosis.

There are two forms of renal metabolic acidosis, which include proximal renal tubular acidosis and distal renal tubular acidosis.

When a person has chronic kidney disease, distal renal tubular acidosis is the most common form of renal metabolic acidosis. This condition transpires when a person's kidneys fail to adequately remove acid from the blood and into the urine. This failure results in an overabundance of acid buildup in the blood. As the blood becomes overly acidic, it can lead to electrolyte imbalances as well as interference with necessary cellular function. Renal tubular acidosis, more broadly referred to as renal metabolic acidosis, can also be shortened and referred to as RTA.

Chemical reactions are , being used throughout the human body to carry out various functions, such as repairing tissue and transforming food into energy. These chemical reactions naturally produce various acids. While some acid is normal and healthy for a balanced blood pH, too much acid results in acidosis, interfering with bodily functions in the process. Thankfully, most people have healthy kidneys that are capable of maintaining a balanced level of acid. It does this by dumping excess acid into urine and delivering alkaline substances, such as bicarbonate, into the bloodstream. This bicarbonate neutralizes acid, balancing the pH of your bloodstream as the acid is created from the process of creating energy.

When RTA is left untreated, it can cause chronic kidney disease, kidney stones, intrauterine growth restriction where a fetus does not develop at a healthy rate, bone disease, and eventually even total kidney failure.

While renal acidosis is rather dangerous if left untreated, it is thankfully simple to diagnose. If you or your doctor suspect you might have RTA, then your doctor can check with simple urine and blood tests. These tests will likely result in a positive diagnosis if the urine is less acidic than normal, and the blood is more acidic than it should be. Although there could be other explanations, only your doctor will be able to know for sure and confirm a diagnosis. Your doctor may want some additional information to rule out any other potential problems. There are a variety of types of RTA, and to determine your type your doctor will run tests on your potassium, chloride, and sodium levels in the urine, as well as potassium levels in your blood. No matter the type of RTA you have, the goal of treatment will be to neutralize the excessive acid in your bloodstream. However, additional treatment measures may need to be taken depending on the type of RTA and the underlying cause of acidosis.

Clinical Types of RTA

Type One, Classical Distal RTA:

Typed One of RTA is named after the location of the defect causing the disorder. "Distal" refers to the location of the problem being distant from where fluid from your blood enters the tubule that collects waste and fluid to produce urine.

There are many causes of this form of RTA, such as the rejection of a transplanted kidney, renal medullary cystic disease, autoimmune disease, hyperparathyroidism, repeated urinary tract infections, and more. Many of these conditions also result in a build-up of calcium deposits in the kidney, triggering impaired distal tubule function in the kidneys. Type One frequently causes low blood potassium levels, which can become extremely dangerous if left untreated. When potassium levels become dangerously low in the bloodstream, it can cause severe weakness, irregular heartbeat, paralysis, and in extreme cases, even death.

When Type One is left untreated, it can result in progressive kidney disease and bone disease, along with interfering with fetal growth. During treatment, the main goals are correcting blood pH and preventing kidney stones. When treated with sodium citrate or sodium bicarbonate, all of the problems tend to be corrected. This will also reduce kidney stone development, stabilize kidney function, and prevent renal failure progression.

Type Two, Proximal RTA:

Type two is named "proximal" RTA as the word means that the defect occurs near the point where waste and fluid from the bloodstream enter the kidney tubule. Type two most frequently occurs in children due to Fanconi's syndrome. Although, it can also be the result of the rare disease cystinosis, inherited disorders, and the use of the chemotherapy drug ifosfamide.

Type Three:

While there was previously a type three, it is no longer used as it is now believed to be a combination of Type One and Type Two.

Type Four, Hyperkalemic RTA:

Type Four is caused by a transport abnormality located in the distal tubule. This abnormality impairs the transport of electrolytes such as potassium, sodium, and chloride, which usually transport through the distal tubule. Type Four is district from types One and Two as it results in high blood potassium levels, rather than low levels. While low potassium levels are dangerous, as we previously mentioned, high levels of potassium are equally as dangerous. Since potassium affects heart health and function, abnormalities of either lows or highs can result in potentially deadly effects if left untreated.

Type Four is caused by problems relating to the hormone aldosterone. When either the kidneys do not properly respond to this hormone or when the blood levels are abnormally low, the kidneys become unable to regulate electrolytes in your blood. Type Four can also develop when the tubule transport of electrolytes is impaired by the use of certain medications or inherited disorders.

Type Four may also develop as a result of another disease that affects kidney function and structure. This includes conditions such as kidney transplant rejection, diabetic nephropathy, urinary tract obstruction, lupus, sickle cell disease, HIV/AIDS, and destruction or removal of both adrenal glands.

If Type Four is treated early, most individuals with the condition will not develop permanent kidney failure. This means that the goal should be early recognition, diagnosis, and treatment. This treatment will need to be maintained and monitored throughout the person's lifespan.

Diagnosis and Treatment

There are different symptoms of renal metabolic acidosis, and not everyone will even experience symptoms. This can make it hard to diagnose, as you if you don't know to look for a problem diagnosis is unlikely. However, as acidosis is a common problem occurring in those with chronic kidney disease, you and your doctor will know to watch out for its development. Your doctor can easily monitor you at set intervals to ensure you do not currently have the disorder or develop it in the future.

While symptoms are not necessary in order to have this disorder, you do want to watch out for the following symptoms, which people may experience in some cases:

- Rapid heart rate

- Deep long breaths

- Rapid breathing

- Weakness

- Fatigue

- Headaches

- Confusion

- Excessive sleepiness

- Loss of appetite

- Nausea

- Vomiting

If you do have chronic kidney disease and metabolic acidosis, there are some increased risks you will have to watch out for, which includes bone loss, muscle loss, endocrine disorders, and progression of the disease. Let's have a quick look at each of these complications in turn.

Bone Loss/Osteoporosis:

Osteoporosis means that your bones have become porous, reduced in both quality and density. As this condition worsens, bones are at an increased risk of developing fractures. This condition usually occurs without any warning, and silently worsens overtime until your bones begin to fracture. When a person has osteoporosis, they are at an increased risk of many bone fractures, and frequently it results in fractures of vital bone structure, such as the hips and spine.

Muscle Loss:

An important protein in your body, albumin, is essential in order to build and maintain healthy muscles. Yet, metabolic acidosis causes low levels of albumin production, leading to what is medically known as muscle wasting or muscle loss.

Endocrine Disorders

The endocrine system is the body's collection of glands that produce hormones. When a person develops metabolic acidosis, it interferes with the function of the endocrine system, potentially affecting many different hormones. For instance, it may cause the development of insulin resistance, resulting in high blood sugar and eventually, diabetes. There are many different endocrine disorders that affect various hormones, and metabolic acidosis can cause various types.

Kidney Disease Progression:

Metabolic acidosis can cause chronic kidney disease, and other kidney diseases, to worsen. Exactly how this occurs is not quite clear. However, it is known that while acid builds up in the bloodstream, the function of the kidneys is reduced, and vice versa, as the kidney function is reduced the acid also further increases. This is why metabolic acidosis can both cause kidney disease and be a symptom of the disease. The longer metabolic acidosis goes on untreated, the more quickly a person's kidney disease will progress, potentially leading to kidney failure.

Treatment:

Bicarbonate plays vital biological functions, as it is a form of carbon dioxide found in our blood. When a person develops low levels of blood bicarbonate, it is a sign of likely metabolic acidosis. This is because bicarbonate is alkaline, meaning it neutralizes the acid. This helps the bloodstream to maintain a healthy pH level, preventing the blood from becoming overly acidic, therefore allowing you to avoid metabolic acidosis. When a person has healthy kidney function, they are able to naturally maintain balanced levels of bicarbonate in their blood. However, this can be obstructed when kidneys are malfunctioning. When a person has less than twenty-two mmol/l of bicarbonate in their blood, it is classified as low bicarbonate, which will cause kidney disease and metabolic acidosis to worsen.

Thankfully, several studies on metabolic acidosis have found that treatment with either sodium citrate or sodium bicarbonate supplements can help to balance blood bicarbonate levels, treat metabolic acidosis, and prevent kidney disease from worsening. However, you should never take this unless your doctor directs you to. This is because it will directly affect your blood's pH, which should be maintained naturally. If you take sodium bicarbonate or sodium citrate when it is not needed, it will negatively affect the pH. Your doctor will be able to run the necessary blood and urine tests to know whether or not you need this treatment, which will ensure that you only benefit your blood's pH and that you don't negatively affect it.

Chapter 5: Protein and Its Influence

The human body requires fuel in order to provide energy for our cells. The three fuel sources in food consist of protein, carbohydrates, and fat. After these are eaten, the digestion system breaks them down into more pure forms of energy, including amino acids from protein, glucose from carbohydrates, and fatty acids from fat. The human body is capable of surviving without consumption of carbohydrates/glucose, as it is capable of transmuting other sources of fuel into any glucose the calls might need in a process known as gluconeogenesis. However, the same is not true of amino acids and fatty acids. There are certain types of amino acids and fatty acids that the human body requires, but is unable to produce on its own. This means that we must consume these fatty acids and amino acids in our diet.

The protein, or amino acids, are used by your body in order to repair damaged tissue, replace old tissues, build muscle, and fight off infections. Thankfully, most people are able to consume protein in the required ranges with neither too much or too little without much effort. As long as they eat a few protein-rich ingredients daily, they can achieve the correct amount of protein. The same is not true of people with kidney diseases, who have to be more diligent in managing how much protein they do or don't consume in their diet.

When a person consumes too much protein, it can cause a buildup of excess waste in their blood. As you know, kidney disease results in the kidneys being unable to properly filter the blood, resulting in excess waste buildup. This means that if a person consumes too much protein when they have kidney disease, they will only be worsening the problem of waste overabundance, and their kidneys will not be capable of handling it. Therefore, it is imperative that people with kidney disease are aware of the amount of protein they consume and that they don't put more than necessary in their meals.

How much protein exactly should you eat if you have been diagnosed with chronic kidney disease? This amount will vary from person to person. This is because the amount of protein a person's body requires to repair cells, build muscle, and fight infection all depends on the person's body size, specific kidney function, and how much protein is being excreted in the urine. Since it is important to avoid either too high or too low protein intake, it is imperative that you discuss this matter with your doctor. Your doctor will be able to calculate your protein requirements with all of your individual elements in mind.

Without amino acids, the body would be incapable of fighting off infections, healing from injuries, and halting excessive bleeding. We would be unable to have any muscle, as well, which would be deadly as the human heart is a muscle itself. This is why it is important to maintain adequate protein intake in your diet. For an average person, protein between forty and sixty-five grams daily is ideal.

Yet, the same is now true of people with kidney disease. A person with chronic kidney disease must be able to limit their protein intake to limit excess waste in the bloodstream and take a burden off the kidneys from filtering said waste. But this must be done while still maintaining their needed protein levels for the body to function. This is why it is important to work together with your doctor to understand your nutrition needs. If you put in the work, understand what to eat, and how much to eat of various nutrients, you can greatly benefit your renal health. Now only do the kidneys manage the waste produced by excess kidneys, but they also filter the other minerals and nutrients you consume. If you eat well, you can take a burden off of your kidneys and consume nutrients that will promote further kidney health. On the other hand, if a person does not watch their diet when they have chronic kidney disease, the results can be disastrous. It can result in loss of appetite, weakness, nausea, taste changes, and overall worsening of the disease.

There are two types of protein you will consume in your daily diet, which are animal-based proteins and plant-based proteins. A person can choose to consume either a combination of both animal and plant proteins or solely plant-based proteins if they are vegan.

Animal-based proteins are simple to add to your diet, as they contain all of the amino acid building blocks your body requires. This means all you have to worry about is consuming the correct amount of protein. The amount and types of fat found within animal-based protein varies based on the source of the ingredient. For example, steak contains much more fat than chicken breasts. Some animal-based proteins are also higher in saturated fats, which are less a less healthy option for heart health. When trying to consume low-saturated fat options for optimal heart health, people typically choose poultry, fish, and reduced-fat dairy options.

Plant-based sources of protein are more versatile in the amino acids they contain. While animal-based proteins contain all the essential amino acids humans require, the variety of amino acids found in most plant-based ingredients is usually reduced. For this reason, if you are relying on plant-based proteins, you will need to ensure you are consuming all nine essential amino acids, which include:

1. lysine

2. isoleucine

3. histidine

4. leucine

5. valine

6. threonine

7. phenylalanine

8. methionine

9. tryptophan

While there are twenty types of amino acids in all, these nine are the most essential to consume in our diets. For this reason, whenever an ingredient contains all nine essential amino acids, it is classified as a complete source of protein. While animal-based products are complete sources of protein, not all plant-based ingredients are. Thankfully, there are still complete sources of plant-based protein, which are important to know about if you are consuming most or all of your protein from plant-based sources. Some examples of complete sources of protein include quinoa, soy, buckwheat, rice paired with beans, and chia seeds. While these are complete sources of protein, you can still get additional amino acids from nuts, grains, lentils, beans, seeds, and vegetables. If a person plans their plant-based diet carefully, they can ensure that they are consuming the correct amount of protein needed for their kidney health and the correct amino acids. Plant-based protein sources are also beneficial as they are low in saturated fat, high in fiber, and high in nutrients.

When consuming protein, you also must consider the minerals found within the protein source. Phosphorus is a mineral that commonly results in a buildup in the blood as kidneys fail to function well. This buildup causes further damage to the kidneys and the body and is therefore often limited. Protein sources that are high in phosphorus include cheese, yogurt, milk, nuts, seeds, beans, peas, peanuts, and soy.

If you have chronic kidney disease and are *not* on dialysis, you will need to limit your protein intake. This is because the more excess waste in your bloodstream, the more effort your kidneys will have to put into working to remove the waste. This causes unnecessary strain on your kidneys, causing them to deteriorate more rapidly. Studies have found that for individuals with chronic kidney disease, who are not on dialysis, it is beneficial to limit protein intake and when you are consuming protein it is generally best to consume plant-based sources rather than animal-based. By making these changes, you can care for your body and reduce the rate of disease progression, better preserving your kidneys.

For patients who have chronic kidney disease and *are* on dialysis, protein needs are different. This is because when a person is on dialysis, it is important to maintain an increased level of protein consumption to maintain needed blood protein levels. As dialysis removes waste from protein from the blood, you no longer have to worry about a low-protein consumption.

Again, the exact amount of protein you need to consume will vary from person to person. Your doctor or nutritionist will determine how much protein you need depending on the stage of your chronic kidney disease, whether or not you are on dialysis, height, weight, and nutrition. Since too much protein can result in kidney deterioration, and too little can result in malnutrition, it is important to follow the amount suggested by a renal-specialized nutritionist or your doctor. Even during the earliest stages of chronic kidney disease, it is important to manage your protein intake carefully.

While the exact amount of protein you will need to consume will vary based on the factors we have previously mentioned, frequently people who are in stages one through three of chronic kidney disease are recommended twelve to fifteen percent of their calorie intake to be protein. If a person is in stage four of chronic kidney disease, this percentage is further reduced, often to being around ten percent of a person's daily caloric intake.

Once a person is diagnosed with chronic kidney disease, one of their first priorities should be discussing their diet with a renal dietitian who can calculate their specific protein requirements. This dietitian or nutritionist can also help customize your diet in other areas, which can be especially beneficial for patients who also have high blood pressure, diabetes, or other conditions common in kidney disease patients.

In general, when a person is prescribed a reduced protein diet for their kidney health, they will eat much smaller portions of protein than they are used to. For instance, they may only eat four to six ounces of animal-based protein daily.

Americans are used to enjoying large servings of protein-rich ingredients, such as meat, fish, and dairy. This can lead to confusion as what you *can* eat if you have to limit these ingredients to such a degree. This is especially confusing when you consider the fact that you must consume enough calories daily to prevent excessive weight loss and muscle waste. Thankfully, there are healthy ingredients that you can add to your meals to increase their nutrition and bulk up calories. One easy way to do this is to add olive oil or avocado oil to your meals. These two oils are high in some of the healthiest fatty acids and are high in calories, allowing a person to easily bulk up their calorie content.

Studies have found that it is frequently beneficial for chronic kidney disease patients to consume more plant-based protein sources rather than animal-based proteins. This means that you can consume more tofu, beans, and grains. The great news is that these studies have found that eating plant-based protein sources for kidney disease patients, rather than animal-based proteins, can greatly increase overall health and reduce death rates.

This study found that for each third of a person's overall protein intake that is from plant-based sources, the person experiences significant improvements. These patients with chronic kidney disease experienced a significantly reduced rate of death, proving the benefits in choosing plant-based ingredients over animal-based ingredients. The researchers concluded that plant-based protein sources could play a vital role in the health outcomes in people with kidney disease.

The exact cause for this improvement with plant-based proteins has not been confirmed. However, there are multiple factors that could be responsible. First, plant-based ingredients are often high in phytonutrients and antioxidants, which have been shown to fight disease and improve overall health. Second, the consumption of these ingredients seems to reduce the production of uremic toxins, which are a type of toxin that is known to worsen the progression of chronic kidney disease and cardiovascular disease.

The third cause of this benefit could lie in the consumption of phosphorus. This mineral, which is known to become overly concentrated in the blood of chronic kidney disease patients, is found in both plant-based and animal-based protein sources. However, the difference is that phosphorus has a different bioavailability rate in both of these sources. While the phosphorus found in animal-based proteins are easily absorbed by the body, the same is not true of plant-based protein sources. This means that a diet that prioritizes plant-based proteins can result in less of a burden of phosphorus on the kidneys.

Chapter 6: Mineral Overload

There are many vital functions of the kidneys, such as filtering out waste from the bloodstream, strengthening bones, and producing red blood cells. Even with these important jobs, there is still another vital function of the kidneys, which is managing the number of minerals in your bloodstream. To do this, as your kidneys filter your blood, they will either pass minerals back through into the bloodstream to be used by the body, or they will expel excess minerals through the urine.

Although, when a person develops chronic kidney disease or kidney failure, then the organs are unable to properly maintain this job well. This frequently results in people with kidney disease also developing mineral and bone disorder, a condition in which a person has an unhealthy imbalance of minerals. This frequently affects phosphorus and calcium, which will affect a person's heart, blood vessels, bones, and more.

When kidneys are unable to function fully, they are no longer able to filter out all of the excess phosphorus in the bloodstream. As this continues to build up over time as you continue to consume phosphorus in your diet, it will result in health problems from the over-concentration.

Your phosphorus and calcium levels will further become out of balance due to your vitamin D levels.

This is because your kidneys are what change vitamin D from the food you eat and the sunlight your skin absorbs into an active form of the vitamin that can be utilized by the body. However, when kidneys function poorly, there is a reduced supply of vitamin D, which influences the phosphorus and calcium balance in your bloodstream.

When a person has too little vitamin D and too much phosphorus in their system, the body will begin to make too much of the parathyroid hormone. When this hormone is overly high, it causes calcium to leech from your bones and into the bloodstream. The result of this is bones that become more brittle and weaker as they lose their needed calcium, causing them to more easily fracture and break. Some of the calcium that leeches out of the bones may also end up in the blood vessels and heart, thereby worsening or causing heart disease.

If you suspect you may have developed mineral and bone disorder, which most chronic kidney disease patients develop, you should talk with your doctor. You should also watch for these symptoms, alerting your doctor to any that you are experiencing:

- Bone pain

- Itchy skin

- Easy bone fractures and breaks

- Anemia

- Heart difficulties

- Blocked blood vessels

- Difficulty fighting germs

In order to test for mineral and bone disorder, your doctor can check your blood levels for vitamin D, calcium, phosphorus, and parathyroid hormone. This simple test should give your doctor all the information they require to either confirm or deny a diagnosis. However, there are cases in which a doctor may need to perform a bone biopsy. Your doctor may also desire to check out the stability of your heart health by ordering an echocardiogram of your heart or an x-ray of your abdomen.

Your doctor will be able to plan the exact treatment you need if you receive a mineral and bone disorder diagnosis. This may include treatment of parathyroid hormone levels, high blood phosphorus levels, and other effects. Many treatment plans include the following:

- **Low Phosphorus Diet**

   By reducing phosphorus in the diet, a person can reduce the excess buildup of this mineral in their bloodstream, getting it closer to a healthy range. Phosphorus from meat, dairy, and other animal-based ingredients should especially be limited, as these sources of the mineral are easily absorbed by the body. On the other hand, plant-based sources of phosphorus are not as bioavailable, meaning that your body will not absorb as much.

- **Phosphate Binders**

  Your doctor may prescribe phosphate binders, which are a medication used to decrease the amount of phosphate absorbed in the stomach from food. This can help to reduce high levels of phosphate, ideally returning them to a balanced and healthy level.

- **Calcimimetics**

  Doctors will prescribe Calcimimetics to reduce levels of calcium, phosphorus, and parathyroid hormone levels.

- **Calcium Supplements**

  You should never take these supplements without your doctor's orders, as it could negatively alter your mineral balance if you do not need them. If you have low calcium levels and are interested in calcium supplements, first discuss the option with your doctor.

- **Vitamin D**

  It is vital for the human body to have an active form of vitamin D, but since the kidneys are responsible for making inactive forms of this vitamin active and available for the cells to utilize, most patients with chronic kidney disease develop deficiencies in this vital vitamin.

Your doctor will discuss medication options with you, most likely giving you a prescription for an active form of vitamin D.

- **Surgery**

  Occasionally, when medication is not enough, a person might have to undergo surgery in order to remove a portion of or all of their parathyroid gland. This is used to help get high levels of the parathyroid hormone under control.

Minerals and Their Affects

Now that you have a general understanding of mineral and bone disorder and the treatment options available, let's have a look at specific minerals and their effect on your health when you have chronic kidney disease.

Phosphorus:

Found within your bones, phosphorus is a needed mineral to keep your bones strong and healthy, along with maintaining the health of other aspects of your body. Normally, when kidneys function well, they can remove any excess phosphorus from your bloodstream. However, when a person has chronic kidney disease, and their kidneys are no longer functioning properly, they lose this ability. While phosphorus is healthy and vital in moderation, in excess, it has the opposite effect and causes harm to your body. In excess, phosphorus can cause calcium to be leeched from your bones, causing bone damage.

When both phosphorus and calcium levels are high, it can result in dangerous calcium deposits in the eyes, lungs, blood vessels, and heart. As time goes on, this can increase the risk of stroke, heart attack, and death. Therefore, maintaining a balanced blood level of phosphorus is vital.

Healthy levels of blood phosphorus are 2.5-4.5 mg/dL. Your doctor can easily learn your phosphorus levels by running a quick blood test.

When a patient is on dialysis, their phosphorus levels will be filtered during treatments, resulting in more balanced blood phosphorus levels. However, dialysis patients can' consume all the high-phosphorus foods they want. They will have to limit phosphorus intake between dialysis treatments to prevent a buildup of this mineral during their everyday life.

Phosphorus is naturally high in protein-rich foods, such as meat, dairy, eggs, fish, beans, and nuts. This is one reason as to why protein is limited to the chronic kidney disease diet. When you do have to consume protein, it is generally better to choose plant-based proteins, as the phosphorus in these are not as easily absorbed by the body, meaning it causes less excessive buildup.

Phosphorus is sometimes added into foods, such as in canned ingredients, fast foods, ready to eat meals, bottled drinks, processed meats, and highly processed foods. This form of phosphorus, added in the form of preservatives and additives, is completely absorbed by the body, making it especially dangerous for those with kidney disease. These should be avoided.

If you look at the ingredient label of foods you can find phosphorus additives and preservatives begin with the letters "phos," such as in the following ingredients:

- Tetrasodium pyrophosphate

- Trisodium phosphate

- Sodium tripolyphosphate

- Sodium hexameta-phosphate

- Monosodium phosphate

- Disodium phosphate

- Dicalcium phosphate

- Phosphoric acid

Sodium:

One of the most abundant elements on earth is sodium. While everyone knows that salt is a form of sodium, specifically sodium chloride, there are other forms of sodium that may be in your food, as well. It is important to avoid high levels of sodium when you have chronic kidney disease, so you need to watch out not only for table salt but also hidden forms of sodium.

Sodium is an essential electrolyte in the human body that manages hydration, blood volume, blood pressure, nerve function, muscle contraction, and acid balance. However, it is easy for people with chronic kidney disease to get too much sodium. This is because when a person has malfunctioning kidneys, they are unable to eliminate excess sodium, resulting in a damaging buildup. This excessive level of sodium will increase blood pressure, in turn, causing further damage to the kidneys.

Some other side effects of excessive blood sodium levels include fluid buildup in the lungs, causing shortness of breath; edema swelling in the hands, legs and face; and an enlarged and weak heart, leading to heart failure.

When you have chronic kidney disease, your doctor will monitor your blood pressure and make recommendations about your sodium content accordingly. Your doctor will know you need to reduce your sodium consumption if your blood pressure is steadily high or if you are retaining excess fluid. You will also be asked to consume a low-sodium diet if you are in stage five of the disease and are on dialysis.

If you are placed on a low-sodium diet, you will need to read the nutrition labels of the foods you eat, which will contain the listed sodium content. Highly processed and fried foods, such as French fries and processed meats, regularly contain an excessive amount of sodium. A low-sodium diet is no more than two-thousand or three-thousand milligrams of sodium daily. Your doctor will give you a specific target recommendation based on your individual case.

Potassium:

Another of the vital electrolytes for human health, potassium is a mineral that manages muscle and nerve functioning. Without potassium, the human heart would be unable to beat. This mineral also affects hydration levels, electrolyte balance, and the body's pH level. Potassium blood levels need to be maintained between 3.5-5.5 mEq/L for it to do its job. Either too much or too little potassium can result in dangerous side effects.

Low potassium is rare, as it is in a large number of foods. Healthy kidneys regularly remove excess potassium from the bloodstream. However, when a person has reduced kidney function, they are no longer able to remove enough excess potassium, resulting in high potassium blood levels. This is known as hyperkalemia and is frequently experienced by people in the late stages of chronic kidney disease. Some of the early signs and symptoms of excessive potassium include weakness, nausea, slow heart rate, and numbness.

When your doctor places you on a low-potassium diet, you will need to avoid potassium-rich ingredients, reduce dairy consumption, discard the liquid from canned foods, avoid potassium chloride, and avoid salt substitutes and seasonings that contain potassium.

Calcium:

The most abundant mineral found in the human body is calcium, as the bones and teeth are made up of primarily this mineral. Out of all the calcium in the human body, ninety-nine percent is contained in the teeth and bones, with the remaining one percent being found in soft tissues and the bloodstream. We use this calcium to maintain healthy bones and teeth; manage healthy blood clotting; control muscle movement and contraction; transmit nerve impulses; assist enzyme reactions; and regulate cell division, multiplication, and secretions.

Calcium is found in a variety of foods, much more than just dairy. However, it is not only our consumption of calcium that matters. This is because the parathyroid hormone and vitamin D directly regular the amount of calcium the human body absorbs and how much calcium the kidneys expel. When kidneys are healthy, they transform vitamin D into the hormone calcitriol, which increases calcium absorption.

However, frequently, people with chronic kidney disease have too little vitamin D and too much parathyroid hormone. This, in turn, affects calcium function and absorption. Your doctor will have to run tests to evaluate your calcium, phosphorus, and parathyroid hormone to assess your calcium needs.

If a patient has low-calcium, their doctor might prescribe phosphorus binders, both to increase calcium levels and decrease phosphorus levels. On the other hand, if a person's calcium levels are high, they will be placed on a low-calcium diet. In order to maintain healthy calcium levels, patients are urged to maintain a low-phosphorus diet, as phosphorus will affect your calcium levels.

When consuming high-calcium foods, it is important to ensure they are also low in phosphorus. This means that dairy is not an option, as it is naturally high in phosphorus.

- Sometimes, grain-products such as crackers and bread may have added calcium, which can be beneficial.

- Bone-in sardines are high in calcium and omega-3 fatty acids.

- Lentils and beans are high in calcium, although they are also high in phosphorus. Thankfully, the phosphorus found in plant-based proteins isn't fully absorbed by the body, making it a better choice than animal-based proteins such as dairy and meat.

- Raw figs are a great option to increase calcium intake without excessive.

- Like beans, tofu is a better protein source than animal-based protein. It is also high in calcium, though you can't eat too much due to the phosphorus content.

- Rhubarb is low in phosphorus while also being high in calcium.

Lastly, remember to work closely with your doctor and renal dietitian. While following the kidney disease diet can greatly help, your doctor and dietitian will always be there if you have any problems. This is helpful, as they can track your mineral levels in your blood, ensuring that if you have either low or high levels that you can make adjustments. If you are unable to maintain your mineral levels through diet alone, your doctor may prescribe medications or supplements.

Chapter 7: The Importance of a Healthy Lifestyle and Diet

I am sure you have heard the phrase, "You are what you eat." But it is not just what you eat that affects your health, but your entire lifestyle. Everything, including your dietary, exercise, medication, drinking, smoking, and sleep habits affect your health. There are other aspects of your lifestyle that can impact your health; this is only the tip of the iceberg. In this chapter, we will be focusing on the importance of a healthy lifestyle, both in treating and preventing chronic kidney disease.

When you have chronic kidney disease, it is incredibly important to focus on promoting healthy lifestyle factors. You can't just take some medicine and get better. Instead, you have to prioritize eating a low-protein diet with the correct proportions of nutrients, exercising to maintain healthy muscles and organs, and sleeping well so that your body has the strength to function to the best of its ability. In one study on chronic kidney disease, it was found that patients who eat a healthy diet, stay physically active, maintain healthy body weight, and don't smoke are able to greatly increase their longevity. The participants who met all of these healthy lifestyle qualities reduced their risks of dying from the disease by sixty-eight percent compared to those who don't follow these lifestyle choices.

These same lifestyle factors have also long been shown to greatly affect heart health and diabetes, which two-thirds of the population with chronic kidney disease also have. This is important to consider, because if your diabetes or heart health is not under control, then it will put more pressure on your kidneys and increase your risk of fatality. On the other hand, if you treat these conditions through a healthy lifestyle, you can greatly improve not only your diabetes or heart health but also your kidney health. Overall, you can only benefit from focusing on improving your lifestyle.

Early Diagnosis:

If you don't yet have chronic kidney disease, but you or a family member are at risk of developing the condition, you can reduce your risk and potentially prevent yourself from developing the disease by making healthy lifestyle changes. Remember, you are more likely to develop kidney disease if you have a family history, diabetes, heart disease, or high blood pressure. If any of these apply to you or someone you love, then consider making the beneficial lifestyle changes mentioned in this chapter.

By managing the conditions associated with kidney diseases, such as diabetes and high blood pressure, you can not only benefit your kidney health but the health of your entire body and mind. In order to maintain a healthy body, it is important that you maintain frequent checkups with your doctor. The frequency of these checkups will depend on your age and any preexisting conditions, and your doctor will be able to recommend a checkup schedule. For people who are in good health, a once-yearly checkup is usually enough. However, if you have any preexisting conditions such as high blood pressure and diabetes, you will need more frequent checkups.

When having your checkup, ask your doctor about monitoring your kidney health. If you are concerned about having a high risk of developing this disease in the future, then your doctor should easily be able to monitor your condition with just a quick urine and blood test at your regular checkups. Your doctor will also keep an eye on your blood sugar and blood pressure to check for diabetes and heart problems. Remember, early diagnosis and treatment is your best option. The earlier you receive a diagnosis for the occurrence of chronic kidney disease, the less risk you will be at of developing dangerous side effects or kidney failure.

If you develop a urinary tract infection, which is rather common, you need to contact your doctor immediately. The infection itself is not dangerous when treated. However, if left untreated, a urinary tract infection can cause chronic damage to your kidneys, potentially causing chronic kidney disease in the future. Thankfully, your doctor can easily prescribe you medicine to treat the infection, which should relatively quickly and prevents unnecessary damage to your kidneys.

Control Your Blood Pressure:

One of the biggest steps you can take to improving your kidney health is managing your blood pressure. Most people only think about the effect blood pressure has on the heart, but it also affects other organs, such as your kidneys. When blood pressure is chronically high, it causes damage to the kidneys. Therefore, you should maintain blood pressure at the goal set by your physician. Most people should aim at blood pressure less than 140/90, as anything over this is considered high.

Blood pressure can become high for different reasons. Therefore, you should discuss a plan with your doctor in order to lower your blood pressure. In general, lowering blood pressure can involve:

- Increased exercise

- Enough sleep

- Higher quality sleep

- Healthy meals with reduced sodium

- Quit smoking

- Taking prescribed medications

Manage Your Blood Glucose:

If you have diabetes, you need to regularly check your blood glucose levels, as prescribed by your doctor. You can use the results you receive in order to make better choices about exercise, food, and medication.

Your doctor will also test your A1C to measure your average blood glucose over the previous three months. The higher your A1C number, then the higher your standard blood glucose levels were during the three-month period. It is important to stay on top of managing your blood glucose and hitting the target blood glucose score given to you by your doctor to meet your A1C goal in the future. Each person is given their own A1C goal by their doctor, but usually, this goal is below seven percent.

By reaching your A1C goal, you can protect your kidney health.

Maintain Low Cholesterol:

High cholesterol runs in families, and it is common in people who make poor lifestyle choices, such as eating an unhealthy diet. This is important to manage, as high cholesterol increases your risk of both heart disease and kidney disease. It is also possible for chronic kidney disease to increase a person's cholesterol. Thankfully, studies have shown that treatment for high cholesterol in patients with chronic kidney disease is the same as those without the disease. This means you can make common-sense changes to improve your cholesterol health, which will be effective even if you have been diagnosed with kidney disease.

When attempting to lower high cholesterol or maintain low cholesterol, keep in mind that there is no specific target level of cholesterol that is universal. Instead, your doctor will advise you on your specific cholesterol levels and what you should aim for.

There are a few different types of cholesterol, but the main two ones you will have to worry about are LDL and HDL.

- LDL = Low Density Lipoprotein

- HDL = High Density Lipoprotein

It is important to know that these two forms of cholesterol are not created equally. LDL is dangerous and damaging cholesterol that is frequently referred to as "bad" cholesterol. This cholesterol increases your risk of heart attack, stroke, and other complications. On the other hand, HDL is frequently known as "good" cholesterol. While LDL cholesterol will cause you harm, HDL cholesterol is beneficial and actually actively lowers LDL cholesterol.

When your doctor measures your cholesterol, they will give you both an LDL and an HDL score. It is actually beneficial to have a high HDL score, although you want your LDL score to be as low as possible.

Foods that are high in cholesterol are typically red meat, dairy products, and eggs, which should be limited to the kidney disease diet, anyways. You will also want to avoid other sources of saturated fats, and instead, use healthy unsaturated fats such as olive oil and avocado oil. By eating a healthy diet with plenty of fruits and vegetables, healthy fats, and reduced intake of saturated fats, you should be able to make great strides in lowering your cholesterol.

Reduce Stress:

When you experience long-term stress, it greatly affects your health. Not only does stress often increase poor life choices, such as smoking, drinking, irregular sleep, and unhealthy diet. But, chronically high stress increases blood sugar, raises blood pressure, and may lead to depression. To manage your stress, you first need to prioritize a healthy lifestyle overall. Exercise, eating well, sleep, and other healthy lifestyle factors can all reduce chronic anxiety. However, you may need other methods of stress relief, as well. Try making a list of any calming activities you find helpful, such as listening to music, meditation, yoga, sketching, reading, or whatever else comes to mind. You can then use this list as inspiration when you are anxious. Whenever you find your stress increased, try completing one or two calming tasks from your list.

Keep in mind that anxiety and depression disorders are common in people experiencing long-term or chronic illnesses. If you are unable to overcome your depression or anxiety on your own, then you may need medical intervention. Try talking to your doctor, who may recommend therapy, anti-anxiety medication, or anti-depressants.

Limit Alcohol Consumption:

By drinking too much, you can negatively raise your blood pressure and consume too many calories, which can cause weight gain and kidney damage. While there can be some benefits to drinking in moderation (unless otherwise instructed by your doctor), you should never exceed the daily recommendation. It is recommended for women to consume no more than one drink daily, and men to consume no more than one or two. The exact amount "one drink" consists of varies depending on the type of alcohol you are drinking. One drink is either 1.5 ounces of heavy liquor, 5 ounces of wine, or 12 ounces of beer.

Quit Smoking:

There is no amount of smoking that is healthy. Smoking only increases your risk of cancer, causes organ damage, raises blood pressure, and increases the risk of heart attack or stroke. Smoking also increases kidney damage. Therefore, it is best to try to quit smoking altogether.

Maintain a Healthy Weight:

Excessive body weight causes your kidneys to push harder in order to complete their work and cause damage over time. Not only that, but excess weight also increases your risk of high blood pressure, high blood sugar, and more. All of these aspects together worsen kidney health, making it vital to maintain a healthy body weight in order to increase kidney health.

Healthy body weight varies greatly from person to person, with BMI (body-mass index) being an unreliable measuring system. Therefore, you should talk to your doctor about your ideal body weight. Thankfully, as you attain a healthy lifestyle, as described in this chapter, you will likely lose weight naturally as all of these factors work together to improve your overall health and weight.

Sleep Well:

Adequate sleep and good sleep quality are important for overall physical and mental health. When you don't sleep well, it can negatively affect you in many ways, such as raising blood pressure and blood glucose. Studies have shown that adults should get seven to eight hours of solid sleep a night.

If you have trouble sleeping, either due to insomnia, sleep apnea, snoring, or poor sleep hygiene, you should see a sleep specialist. This specialist can make sure you don't have any hidden sleep disorders preventing you from sleeping well or soundly, and they can create a schedule for optimal sleep hygiene.

Exercise Regularly:

It is best to try to be active for at least thirty minutes a day. However, you should specifically try to maintain thirty minutes of moderate exercise three to four times a week. Along with with moderate exercise, it is a good idea to also include some light flexibility-based exercises, which can reduce your risk of injury and make your more difficult exercises easier.

While you can always workout at a gym, you can also simply walk around the block, lift some small weights at home, and practice yoga stretches in your living room. Of course, it is also a good idea to include a variety of exercise as you are able, to work out a larger portion of your body.

Be Careful of OTC Medications:

Of course, you should take any prescribed medication your doctor gives you. Speaking of, whenever you see any of your doctors make sure that they all know every single medication you are taking, whether prescribed or over-the-counter, as well as supplements. These can affect your health in more ways than you might realize, and a simple over-the-counter supplement could negatively interact with one of your conditions or medications.

Along with giving your doctor a list of your medications, you should also talk to either your doctor or pharmacist before taking any new over-the-counter medications or supplements. These can cause many problems, which might not be listed on the label. For instance, many painkillers can damage the kidneys and should not be taken by anyone with kidney disease or injury.

As you know, diet is also an important aspect of your lifestyle. However, we will discuss the details of the kidney disease diet in a later chapter, so stay tuned!

Chapter 8: New Therapies, Cures, and Medicines for Kidney Disease

In this chapter, we will explore some of the newest scientifically discovered therapies, cures, and medicines for kidney disease. Some of these are currently on the market, others will soon be available, and others yet are still in the early stages of development. While all of these might not be quite yet available at this time, they have shown amazing results or promise, and offer more hope for the future. For those treatment options that are available, if you are interested in whether or not they will work in your case, you should consult on the matter with your doctor.

Recently, the National Kidney Foundation joined together with the European Medicines Agency and the Food and Drug Administration to hold a joint scientific workshop. During this time, these organizations reviewed the largest compilation of multi-year meta-analysis on chronic kidney disease to date. The data was so extensive that it included nearly two-million participants, meaning that the results are more trustworthy and sounder. During their review, they found evidence supporting the use of early markers in the detection and monitoring of kidney disease. This means that there can soon be new treatments that can treat people with chronic kidney disease. One of the main goals of the scientific community at this time is to find new treatment options that can be used in early-stage kidney disease, to prevent it from progressing to the end stage of the disease. By doing this, it would allow people to receive treatment without degrading to the point where they require transplantation or dialysis.

Some of the elements that the researchers were analyzing during this workshop were whether changes in the albumin protein found in urine and glomerular filtration rate could be used as predictors of how effective treatment could be.

During the course of the workshop, much important research was shared, allowing for better research and treatment options in the future. This is wonderful news, as more treatment options to reduce the progression and risk of chronic kidney disease have been needed.

Often times, people with chronic kidney disease experience protein leakage from the kidneys, which is known as proteinuria. This, in turn, worsens the kidney disease, resulting in further damage to the organs. Although, a new breakthrough drug therapy might be able to alleviate the damage, this side effect causes.

This drug therapy uses a blocker compound that is combined with another one that is also used in the treatment of high blood pressure and nephropathy in patients with type II diabetes. One of the researchers for the study explained that these specific blocker compounds are being used, as it was found that they have a beneficial interaction with the receptors in the kidney cells that they bind onto.

There has been recent hope for patients with both chronic kidney disease and type II diabetes, which is wonderful news considering that nearly half of the individuals with kidney disease also have diabetes. In a trial on a new medication, canagliflozin, it was found that this medication could offer new hope in reducing the progression of the disease. This is the first time in over fifteen years that success such as this has been achieved.

During the course of the trial, four-thousand and four-hundred individuals with both chronic kidney disease and type II diabetes participated. The canagliflozin, also sold under the brand name Invokana, showed such amazing results and proved safe so quickly that the trial was able to end sooner than expected.

While there are some medications that lower blood pressure and reduce the risk of chronic kidney disease, these other medications are only partially effective. On the other hand, Invokana, a small daily pill meant to control blood sugar, has been shown to be much more effective in preventing chronic kidney disease and reducing the risk of kidney failure. The study found that the participants on Invokana experienced a thirty percent reduced risk of kidney failure, the need for dialysis treatment, required kidney transplantation, or death related to either kidney or heart problems.

Worldwide, there are one hundred and sixty million people with type II diabetes who are at risk of also developing chronic kidney disease. With this new medication option on the horizon, it offers new options in preventing the risk of kidney failure, transplantation, and dialysis. The importance of these results cannot be overstated.

With the rise of type II diabetes and chronic kidney disease in the western world, the demand and need for kidney transplantation have also increased. However, there are not enough organ donors to meet this great and increasing need. Thankfully, in the future, there may be more options available for those who would otherwise need a transplant. This is due to the current research and analysis of therapy based on stem cells, which offer an exciting opportunity for the future.

While the results of stem cell research will not be seen by patients for years to come, scientists have found some exciting possibilities. For instance, researchers are currently studying how it is possible for the kidneys to regenerate themselves rather than requiring transplantation. To this end, researchers are attempting to discover which type of kidney cells are needed for the process.

As kidney disease is a result of different cell types being damaged in the kidneys, researchers must consider which cells are damaged. This means that stem cell treatments are only effective when researchers know which cells were damaged and need replacement.

While it is still yet to be clear which type of cells are needed for kidney regeneration, there are several groups of cells that are being investigated. Some of these cells, that are located around the nephrons, possess characteristics similar to stem cells. One of the cell groups currently being investigated is the renal progenitor cells. There is another type of cell that is also being investigated, which is similar to the cells found in bone marrow, known as mesenchymal stem cells.

One type of stem cell being used in ongoing research is the pluripotent stem cells. These cells are being used to create 3D structures similar to the nephrons of our kidneys. The purpose of this is to analyze how they are formed in embryos, test new drug therapy options, and create the possibility of replacing the nephrons on damaged kidneys in the future.

While there are studies on stem cells in the treatment of chronic kidney disease, another study is taking a different approach. In this study, rather than studying stem cells themselves, they are studying the extracellular vesicle particles that are released by the stem cells. The results, if the research continues to progress well, could offer an alternative treatment option to stem cell therapy.

The human kidneys are truly amazing. Several years back, researchers discovered that they have the ability to regenerate and repair themselves over time. Although, this regeneration process does have its limits. For instance, because many people go undiagnosed with chronic kidney disease due to the lack of symptoms in the early stages, the damage to the kidneys frequently becomes too severe for the kidneys to repair themselves.

It is easy to see why stem cell therapy would be helpful in this case. Yet, the researchers for this study believe that the highest level of potential lies not in stem cells themselves, but instead the extracellular vesicle particles released by stem cells.

The extracellular vesicles otherwise referred to as "EVs," have been found to mimic the cellular biological activity by transporting stem cell-derived molecules to the damaged tissue of the kidneys. The use of EVs rather than stem cells themselves is beneficial, as they do not trigger an immune system reaction, are biocompatible, and they can be administered to patients in the form of a drug.

Some of the benefits of EVs is that they have been shown to inhibit the production of fibrosis tissue, which is harmful to the kidneys and can eventually lead to kidney failure. They have also been shown to trigger the regeneration of the tubular epithelial cells and lead to an overall regenerative effect of the kidneys.

While more studies and research are needed before patients can benefit from EVs in the treatment of chronic kidney disease, the results are incredibly inspiring. In a number of years, it is possible that the damage to kidneys from chronic kidney disease may be reversible.

Chapter 9: Treating Your Kidney Disease with Success

If you hope to successfully treat your chronic kidney disease, then you need to focus on your diet. This means that you should limit your protein, phosphorus, calcium, and sodium intake. Along with this, you should focus on eating a wide variety of healthy foods such as vegetables, fruits, and grains. Ideally, you should prioritize plant-based proteins over animal-based proteins, as the phosphorus in these is absorbed to a lesser degree, helping to reduce the dangerous phosphorus buildup in the bloodstream. In this chapter, we will focus on how you can successfully treat your chronic kidney disease by eating well and making better food choices.

Kidney Disease Diet for Stages One Though Four

When you have chronic kidney disease, it is important to be careful of everything you put in your body, as your kidneys are less able to filter out waste or manage mineral contents in the bloodstream. Therefore, you want to eat in a way that reduces damage to your kidneys as much as possible. During the early stages of kidney disease, you will have more freedoms in what you eat, but as kidney disease progresses, you have to take more precautions.

Ideally, you want to consume a diet high in fruits and vegetables; with healthy fats and grains; some nuts, seeds, and beans; a small amount of protein and dairy; and low in sugar, sodium, phosphorus, magnesium, trans fats, and saturated fats.

Everyone needs protein in their diets. Even if you have chronic kidney disease and have to limit your protein intake, you still need some. This is because protein is used to fight infections, replace damaged cells, and maintain the mass of our muscles (including the heart). But how much protein should you be eating? There is not one standard number, as protein intake varies depending on a person's size, age, sex, and overall health.

There is a Recommended Dietary Allowance for healthy adults, which should be adjusted by a person's doctor if they have a condition such as chronic kidney disease. The recommendation is 0.8 grams of protein for every kilogram of body weight. This means that if an average healthy adult weighs 150, then they should be consuming 55 grams of protein daily to maintain their health requirements. If a person weighs 120 pounds, then they will need 44 grams of protein.

It is important to maintain adequate protein levels, as too little will cause muscle wasting, damage your heart, and result in increased infections. For most people, a slight increase in protein intake is not damaging, as their kidneys can filter out any waste byproducts and excrete them through the urine. However, this ability is diminished in people with chronic kidney disease. As these people have less kidney function, the waste byproducts are unable to be filtered out by the kidneys and result in a buildup of the waste in the bloodstream. This process increases the speed of kidney damage, worsening the disease at a rapid rate. Thankfully, studies have shown that if individuals with chronic kidney disease limit their protein intake, they can also slow the rate of progression of the disease and preserve kidney function.

A kidney specialist, known as a nephrologist, and a renal dietitian will be able to help a person determine how much protein they should consume when they have chronic kidney disease. They can calculate how much protein the body needs to maintain its normal function, while also reducing the protein intake to treat the disease and reduce kidney damage.

When eating protein, it is important to remember the difference between plant-based and animal-based proteins. While animal-based proteins contain all nine essential amino acids, making them a complete protein source, there are benefits to choosing plant-based protein sources instead. First, most sources of animal-based protein contain damaging saturated fats, which are generally not in plant-based proteins.

But, more importantly, phosphorus in plant-based proteins is less bioavailable than the phosphorus in animal-based proteins, which means your body will absorb less, thereby also lessening the damaging buildup of phosphorus in your bloodstream. When possible, choose plant-based protein sources over animal-based protein sources.

While animal-based sources are known as complete protein sources, there are some complete protein sources from plants. These mainly include soy products such as tofu, beans paired with rice, buckwheat, quinoa, and chia seeds. You can also find protein in many vegetables, grains, nuts, seeds, beans, and lentils. These are also high in fiber, which helps to lower blood sugar and cholesterol!

When you do choose animal-based protein sources, the best options that are low in saturated fat are fish, white meat poultry, and low-fat dairy products.

Let's have a look at some ways you can get a daily dose of protein. For this example, the protein requirement will be 50-60 grams, but you will need to discuss your specific protein needs with your doctor.

- Quinoa, cooked - .5 cup

- Yogurt, low-fat - .5 cup

- Beans, cooked - .5 cup

- Chicken breast – 4 ounces

With this example, a person can consume 53 grams of protein over the course of their day. It also contains 707 milligrams of phosphorus, 176 milligrams of sodium, 320 milligrams of calcium, and 1090 milligrams of potassium.

Limit the Sodium, Phosphorus, Potassium, and Calcium:

Sodium is found in many foods; it is more than only table salt. It is important to be careful with this mineral and your consumption of it, especially when you have high blood pressure or chronic kidney disease. This is because sodium affects the water balance in your body and can greatly raise your blood pressure, in the process causing more kidney damage and increasing your risk of heart disease. Thankfully, your doctor can run a simple blood test to see the mineral levels in your bloodstream, which will allow you to know whether or not your sodium levels are too high.

If your blood pressure is at a healthy level, and you are only in the early stages of chronic kidney disease, you can aim for two to three grams of sodium a day. However, if you are in the later stages of kidney disease with high blood pressure, you should reduce your sodium consumption to be below two grams daily.

In order to cut your sodium consumption, you should avoid:

- Table salt

- Sea salt

- Garlic salt

- Seasoning salt

- Soy sauce

- Onion salt

- Celery salt

- Meat tenderizer

- Lemon pepper.

- Oyster sauce

- Teriyaki sauce

- Barbecue sauce

- Cured foods, such as meats and vegetables

- Lunch meats

Most fast foods and highly processed foods are high in sodium, meaning that cooking at home is your best option. This doesn't mean you have to cook difficult and elaborate meals; they can be simple and easy. Since you cannot include salt, instead enjoy a wide selection of sodium-free spices and herbs. Whenever you cook with canned foods, you should drain off the liquid and then rinse the food in warm water, to remove excess sodium. Lastly, always read ingredient labels to check the sodium content.

It is important to watch your phosphorus levels, to prevent a buildup in your bloodstream. Ask your doctor how much phosphorus you should aim for as your daily intake. In general, when a person develops late-stage kidney disease, their doctor will advise them to consume no more than one gram of phosphorus daily.

You can limit your phosphorus intake by limiting dairy consumption, cutting back on meats and fish, reading ingredient and nutrition labels to avoid high phosphorus ingredients, avoiding dark-colored sodas, increasing fresh fruits and vegetables, and consuming more rice and corn products.

Your doctor will likely recommend that you reduce your calcium intake, which shouldn't be difficult as foods high in calcium are generally also high in phosphorus. This means you naturally will not be consuming much calcium. The easiest way to reduce your calcium intake is to limit dairy products, bone-in fish, seeds, and fortified foods.

Lastly, you should limit your potassium intake. This mineral is really important, but most people consume much more than they need. While this is not generally a problem, it becomes one for people with decreased renal function as their kidneys are no longer able to filter out the excess potassium, causing a buildup in the bloodstream. This can be more difficult to avoid, as many foods are rich in potassium, such as fruits and vegetables. In general, you don't want to consume any more than two grams of potassium daily.

Try to limit potassium-rich foods, such as:

- Tomatoes

- Potatoes

- Sweet Potatoes

- Cranberries

- Blueberries

- Strawberries

- Raspberries

- Plums

- Star fruit

- Avocados

- Bananas

- Whole-wheat bread

- Brown rice

- Dairy

- Oranges

- Apricots

- Winter Squash

- Beets

- Dark leafy greens

- Dried fruits

- Parsnips

- Rutabaga

Kidney Disease Diet for
Stage Five and Dialysis Patients

When you are in the fifth stage of chronic kidney disease, in which your kidneys fail and you most likely begin dialysis, you have to take even more precautions than you do in stages one through four of kidney disease. This means that you have to be even more careful in which foods you eat, how much protein you consume, and the number of minerals in your meals.

Since you will now be on dialysis, you will need to limit your fluid intake and foods that cause a buildup of waste or excess minerals int eh bloodstream. Your doctor, renal dietitian, and the dialysis center should be able to help you monitor your diet and answer any questions you might need. These people are important resources to have because even though there may be general guidelines written about in this book, every person is an individual and might need adjustments based on their specific situation. These doctors, dietitians, and nurses are there to help and can help you customize your diet to ideally fit your needs.

If you also have high blood pressure, high cholesterol, or diabetes, you will be happy to know that this diet will not only benefit your chronic kidney disease but your other conditions, as well.

In general, dialysis patients need to:

- Consume more protein-rich foods

- Consume less sodium, phosphorus, and potassium

- Control fluid intake including water, tea, coffee, juices, and other beverages

Fluids:

While many people in today's day and age do not drink enough water, the same is not true of dialysis patients. In fact, people who are undergoing dialysis therapy can easily consume too much water, causing a fluid overload known as hypervolemia. The kidneys are responsible for balancing the amount of fluid in your body, but when this is disrupted is can negatively affect your health, causing swelling and difficulty breathing.

When a person begins dialysis treatment, their kidneys are no longer able to balance the amount of fluid is in their body. This results in them being unable to remove enough fluid, causing a buildup in the body. This is also why you have to be even more vigilant in reducing sodium intake, as sodium affects your body's fluid levels. Thankfully, if you can carefully manage both your fluid and sodium intake, your dialysis treatments should be able to maintain the correct amount of these two in your body, removing any excess.

If you are worried you may have consumed too much liquid you should watch for symptoms of swelling in your hands, feet, and face; shortness of breath; high blood pressure; cramping, headaches, and bloating; and heart problems such as changes in your heart rate or palpitations.

You can better manage your fluid intake by tracking how much you are drinking. Some people may prefer to do this with a small notebook they can keep on them, although it is generally easier to use a smartphone app. There are many apps designed to track your liquid intake. Remember, when tracking your intake don't only track water, but any and all liquid you consume.

You can better manage your thirst by sucking on sugar-free hard candies, frozen grapes, and ice chips. These can help you to avoid drinking too much between your dialysis therapy sessions.

Keep in mind that sodium causes your body to hold onto water. You will have to be even more careful with your sodium intake than you were in earlier stages of kidney disease.

Follow the fluid recommendations given to you by your doctor and dialysis team. This will vary from person to person based on their body and various lifestyle factors. However, most people are instructed to limit their fluid intake to only thirty-two ounces daily.

If you have concerns about developing fluid overload, then have a talk with your healthcare team. They may need to adjust your dialysis treatments to account for any concerns, such as including either longer or more frequent dialysis treatments.

Meat and Protein:

While people in earlier stages of kidney disease need to limit their protein intake, patients in stage five who are on dialysis will be required to increase their protein intake. By increasing your protein, you can maintain healthy blood protein levels and improve your overall health.

Try choosing fish, poultry, and eggs while generally avoiding red meat, which is high in saturated fats. In general, you will want to eat eight to ten ounces of high-protein ingredients, such as meat, dairy.

Beans, lentils, peas, nuts, seeds, and peanuts will have to be eaten in moderation. Keep in mind that these foods are high in phosphorus and potassium, so you should only eat small servings of them when it does not cause you to go over your daily limit.

Grains and Cereals:

Grains and cereals can be a great option, in some cases. Not everyone can enjoy these foods as if you are having trouble managing your blood sugar; they could spike it even more. Therefore, it is generally best for diabetic patients to limit grains.

When choosing grains try to avoid whole-grain or high-fiber varieties, such as brown rice and whole-wheat bread. While these are generally better options for healthy people, the same is not true for those with chronic kidney disease, as they contain a larger amount of phosphorus. Instead, choose the processed forms of grains such as white rice, pasta, and white bread.

Fruits and Vegetables:

When consuming fruits and vegetables, you want to select varieties that are low in phosphorus and potassium. It is helpful that canned fruits are lower in potassium than the fresh alternates. On the other hand, canned vegetables have more sodium and should be rinsed off before using.

It is a good idea to download a diet app on your smartphone and track what you eat. Try to find an app option that will give you the full nutritional details of what you are eating, so that you can easily track your mineral intake and reduce the risk of overconsumption.

Try to consume two or three servings of low-potassium fruits daily, such as:

- Apple – 1

- Pear – .5

- Peach – 1

- Tangerine – 1

- Plums – 2

- Cherries – 10

- Berries - .5 cup

- Fruit cocktail, drained - .5 cup

- Grapes – 15

- Pineapple, canned, drained - .5 cup

- Watermelon, small wedge – 1

Consume two to three servings of low-potassium vegetables daily. Keep in mind that they will all have some potassium, which you need to track so that you aren't consuming more than you believe.

Some options include:

- Cabbage

- Radishes

- Broccoli

- String Beans

- Lettuce

- Eggplant

- Celery

- Watercress

- Peppers

- Cauliflower

- Carrots

- Eggplant

- Yellow Squash

- Zucchini

- Onions

Chapter 10: Recipes

In this final chapter, we will go over some recipes to get you started on a healthy kidney diet! The recipes are divided into two portions, one set for those with types one through four of chronic kidney disease, and one set of recipes for those in type five that are on dialysis. It is important to remember that these two sets are to stay separate, as people in these different stages require different dietary needs.

If you are interested in gaining more recipes for the kidney disease diet, learning meal planning, and more, then look for _The Renal Diet Cookbook_, by the same authors as _Kidney Disease Diet_, Dr. Elizabeth Torres, and Dr. Robert Porter.

Note:
Pictures about medical recipes are Not included within this book.

Dr. Elizabeth Torres used her specialty (dietitian specialised in renal diet) to share recipes specifically for the kidney disease diet, complete with easy to follow
step-by-step instructions and nutritional information.

You will love these recipes, their ease, how they can benefit your health, and their flavor. These recipes are truly delicious, making the kidney disease diet enjoyable.

Types 1-4

Greek Yogurt Pancakes

These pancakes are quick and easy to whip up, perfect for any day of the week! Try topping them with sugar-free syrup or fresh fruit.

The Details:

The Number of Servings: 2

The Time Needed to Prepare: 2 minutes

The Time Required to Cook: 7 minutes

The Total Preparation/Cook Time: 9 minutes

Number of Calories in Individual Servings: 171

Protein Grams: 9

Phosphorus Milligrams: 217

Potassium Milligrams: 240

Sodium Milligrams: 56

Fat Grams: 6

Total Carbohydrates Grams: 19

Net Carbohydrates Grams: 19

The Ingredients:

Eggs, large – 1

Greek yogurt, low-fat - .25 cup

Rice milk – 2 tablespoons

Baking powder, low-sodium - .5 teaspoon

All-purpose flour – 1/3 cup

Olive oil - .5 tablespoon

The Instructions:

1. In a mixing bowl combine together the rice milk, Greek yogurt, and egg with a small whisk.

2. Add the all-purpose flour and low-sodium baking powder to the bowl and whisk until everything is well combined. However, try to avoid mixing the pancake mixture, it is okay if there are small clumps.

3. Heat an electric griddle or a skillet over medium to medium-high heat. Once hot, grease the skillet with the olive oil and pour the pancake batter into small circles on the pan.

4. Allow the pancakes to cook until the dough is full of air bubbles and begins to look dry, then flip them over. Don't mess with the pancakes unless you are flipping them, as it can cause them to stick or break. Once the other side of the pancakes has become golden, remove them from the skillet and cook any leftover batter.

5. Serve the pancakes immediately with your favorite toppings.

Cauliflower Breakfast Hash

This cauliflower hash makes a wonderful alternative to traditional potato hashes, which are too high in potassium to be allowed on the kidney diet. The spices and herbs will also increase the flavor, making this hash one of your favorites! Don't worry about the fat of the olive oil, as it is a source of heart-healthy fat.

The Details:

The Number of Servings: 2

The Time Needed to Prepare: 2 minutes

The Time Required to Cook: 10 minutes

The Total Preparation/Cook Time: 12 minutes

Number of Calories in Individual Servings: 277

Protein Grams: 7

Phosphorus Milligrams: 125

Potassium Milligrams: 304

Sodium Milligrams: 82

Fat Grams: 25

Total Carbohydrates Grams: 7

Net Carbohydrates Grams: 5

The Ingredients:

Cauliflower florets – 1 cup

Eggs – 2

Onion, diced - .25 cup

Bell pepper, diced - .25 cup

Paprika – .5 teaspoon

Cayenne pepper - .25 teaspoon

Cilantro, dried – 1 teaspoon

Cumin – .5 teaspoons

Olive oil – 3 tablespoons

The Instructions:

1. In a small bowl combine the paprika, cayenne pepper, dried cilantro, and cumin before setting the bowl of spices over to the side for later.

2. Place a large non-stick skillet on the stove over a temperature of medium heat. Add in the olive oil, diced bell pepper, diced onion, and cauliflower florets. Allow these vegetables to cook together until they become softened, about five minutes.

3. Sprinkle the prepared cumin and paprika spice mixture over the top of the vegetables and stir them together until completely combined. Place

a lid over the skillet and continue to sauté the vegetables in the olive oil until the cauliflower is fork-tender. Occupational remove the lid to stir the vegetables until they are ready.

4. Remove the lid from the skillet and make two "wells" in the vegetables big enough for the eggs. Crack one egg into each of the weeks, cover the skillet with the lid again, and allow it to cook until the eggs are set. Remove the skillet from the heat and serve the hash immediately.

Chicken Fajita Bowls

This meal is a perfect balance of meat, vegetables, and grains, making it a great option to enjoy for lunch or dinner. You can easily serve this meal immediately, or make it ahead of time and save it in the fridge to take with you to work for lunch.

The Details:

The Number of Servings: 2

The Time Needed to Prepare: 5 minutes

The Time Required to Cook: 15 minutes

The Total Preparation/Cook Time: 20 minutes

Number of Calories in Individual Servings: 365

Protein Grams: 17

Phosphorus Milligrams: 229

Potassium Milligrams: 510

Sodium Milligrams: 46

Fat Grams: 11

Total Carbohydrates Grams: 47

Net Carbohydrates Grams: 45

The Ingredients:

Chicken breast - .25 pound

Olive oil – 1.5 tablespoons

Bell pepper, red – 1

Bell pepper, green – 1

Onion – 1

Garlic, minced – 4 cloves

Chili powder - .25 teaspoon

Cayenne pepper – pinch

Paprika - .25 teaspoon

Cumin - .25 teaspoon

Black pepper, ground - .25 teaspoon

White rice, cooked – 1.5 cups

The Instructions:

1. Combine the chili powder, cayenne pepper, paprika, cumin, and black pepper together to make your fajita seasonings and then set the spices aside.

2. Slice the chicken breast into bite-sized cubes and then place it in a small bowl, massaging it with half of the prepared seasoning mix. Allow it to marinate for fifteen minutes.

3. In a large skillet, with one tablespoon of the olive oil set over medium-high heat cook the

onion and bell pepper until softened, about five minutes.

4. Add in the chicken and garlic, and continue to cook until the chicken is fully cooked through, reaching an internal temperature of Fahrenheit one-hundred and sixty-five degrees. This should take about ten minutes. Don't forget to stir the chicken occasionally.

5. Remove the skillet from the heat and serve the vegetables and chicken over the rice.

Single Pan Balsamic Chicken and Veggies

This chicken and vegetable recipe is incredibly simple, and only requires one pan! You can enjoy it either immediately for a fresh dinner, or save it in the fridge or freezer for an easy lunch during the week.

The Details:

The Number of Servings: 2

The Time Needed to Prepare: 5 minutes

The Time Required to Cook: 15 minutes

The Total Preparation/Cook Time: 20 minutes

Number of Calories in Individual Servings: 346

Protein Grams: 18

Phosphorus Milligrams: 208

Potassium Milligrams: 504

Sodium Milligrams: 89

Fat Grams: 8

Total Carbohydrates Grams: 48

Net Carbohydrates Grams: 45

The Ingredients:

Chicken, breast, cut into bite-sized pieces - .33 pound

Baby carrots – 1 cup

Onion, sliced – 1

Olive oil – 1 tablespoon

Balsamic vinegar – 1 tablespoon

Italian herb seasoning – 1 teaspoon

Black pepper, ground - .25 teaspoon

Garlic, minced – 4 cloves

Rice, white, cooked – 1.5 cups

The Instructions:

1. Preheat your oven to a temperature of Fahrenheit four-hundred degrees before lining a baking tray with kitchen parchment.

2. In a small bowl use a whisk to combine together the olive oil, balsamic vinegar, Italian herb seasoning, black pepper, and minced garlic.

3. Place the bite-sized chicken pieces in a bowl and add in half of the vinegar and seasoning mix, massaging the mixture into the chicken. Allow the chicken to marinate for fifteen to thirty minutes ideally, or use it right away.

4. Place the chicken and vegetables on the pan and toss them in the remaining prepared seasoning and vinegar mixture until evenly coated. Spread the vegetables and chicken out on the pan so

that they cook evenly, and then set the pan into the center of your preheated oven.

5. Cook the mixture for fifteen minutes before turning the pan around to allow for even cooking, and then continue to cook for an additional fifteen minutes. Check and make sure that the chicken has reached an internal temperature of Fahrenheit one-hundred and sixty-five degrees. Remove the pan from the oven if it is ready, and if not allow it to cook for a few more minutes.

6. Serve the vegetables and chicken over rice, either immediately or save them for lunch later in the week.

Pink Salmon with Roasted Broccoli

This salmon and roasted broccoli are delicious and extremely easy! Just keep in mind that the salmon is higher in potassium than poultry. However, as long as you make sure that the meals you eat during the remainder of your day don't put you over your potassium goal, then you should be okay. It is a good thing to include healthy fatty fish, such as salmon, which you can, as it has many health benefits and vital omega-3 fatty acids.

The Details:

The Number of Servings: 2

The Time Needed to Prepare: 5 minutes

The Time Required to Cook: 15 minutes

The Total Preparation/Cook Time: 20 minutes

Number of Calories in Individual Servings: 318

Protein Grams: 21

Phosphorus Milligrams: 301

Potassium Milligrams: 515

Sodium Milligrams: 81

Fat Grams: 11

Total Carbohydrates Grams: 32

Net Carbohydrates Grams: 31

The Ingredients:

Salmon fillets – 6 ounces

Lemon zest - .25 teaspoon

Olive oil – 1 tablespoon

Broccoli florets – 1 cup

Cumin - .25 teaspoon

Lemon juice – 2 teaspoons

Garlic, minced – 2 cloves

Red pepper flakes - .125 teaspoon

Thyme, dried - .25 teaspoon

Rice, white, cooked – 1.25 cups

The Instructions:

1. Preheat your oven to a temperature of Fahrenheit four-hundred and twenty-five degrees and line a baking pan with kitchen parchment.

2. Place the broccoli florets on the baking sheet, drizzle the olive oil over the top, and toss the florets in the oil until they are evenly coated. Spread the florets around the pan.

3. Set the salmon fillets on the baking pan, between the broccoli florets.

4. In a small bowl combine the lemon zest, cumin, lemon juice, garlic, red pepper flakes, and thyme. Spread this mixture over the top of the salmon. Set the pan in the oven and allow it to cook until the salmon is cooked through and flaky, about ten to fifteen minutes.

5. Remove the baking sheet from the oven and serve the rice, vegetables, and fish together. You may want to give a squeeze of fresh lemon over the top of it. It is also nice to add a little extra dried thyme and black pepper to the cooked rice.

Easy and Gourmet Pasta Salad

This pasta salad is full of nutrition, with homemade turkey meatballs, fresh mushrooms and asparagus, and heart-healthy olive oil. Enjoy this dish either immediately after making it, or enjoy it later on as a cold refrigerated treat.

The Details:

The Number of Servings: 2

The Time Needed to Prepare: 5 minutes

The Time Required to Cook: 20 minutes

The Total Preparation/Cook Time: 25 minutes

Number of Calories in Individual Servings: 474

Protein Grams: 22

Phosphorus Milligrams: 257

Potassium Milligrams: 419

Sodium Milligrams: 65

Fat Grams: 11

Total Carbohydrates Grams: 52

Net Carbohydrates Grams: 48

The Ingredients:

Pasta, cooked – 2 cups

Turkey, ground - .25 pound

Italian seasoning – 1 teaspoon

Bread crumbs, plain without seasonings – 1 tablespoon

Black pepper, ground - .25 teaspoon

Garlic minced – 3 cloves

Mushrooms, sliced – .5 cup

Asparagus - .25 pound

Balsamic vinegar – 1 tablespoon

Olive oil – 2 tablespoons

The Instructions:

1. Start boiling a pot of water and cook the pasta according to the directions on the packaging. Meanwhile, preheat a large skillet on the stove over medium heat. Preferably, you want to use a non-stick skillet.

2. While the skillet preheats, combine the ground turkey with the breadcrumbs, black pepper, minced garlic, and half of the Italian seasoning. Be careful not to over mix the meat. Otherwise, it will become tough.

3. Using a spoon scoop out easily-sized portions and then roll them between your hands to form balls. You want each meatball to contain about

two to three teaspoons of meat. A tablespoon contains three teaspoons, meaning that it is a helpful spoon to use to measure out the meat. Just be sure you don't heap the meat over the edge of the tablespoon, or else you will have too much meat mixture.

4. Add one tablespoon of the olive oil to the skillet, add in the rolled meatballs, and cook the meatballs until cooked all the way through with no pink in the center. The middle needs to reach a temperature of Fahrenheit one-hundred- and sixty-five-degrees Fahrenheit. Be sure to stir the meatballs around occasionally so that all sides can cook!

5. Once the meatballs are done cooking remove them from the skillet and set them aside. Add the mushrooms and asparagus to the skillet, allowing them to cook until tender, about seven to nine minutes. Remove the skillet from the heat.

6. In a medium-sized bowl add the cooked pasta, meatballs, and vegetables along with the remaining Italian seasoning, one tablespoon of olive oil, and the balsamic vinegar. Toss all of the ingredients together and serve it warm, or chill it in the fridge before serving.

Greek Chicken Pita Sandwiches

For these pita sandwiches, be sure that you don't use whole-wheat or enriched pita bread, you want to use white pita bread as it is lowest in phosphorus and potassium. When making this recipe, please keep in mind that while this recipe uses onion and garlic powder, these are not the same as garlic and onion salt. These are different ingredients, as the powder contains much less sodium than the salt variety.

The Details:

The Number of Servings: 2

The Time Needed to Prepare: 5 minutes

The Time Required to Cook: 25 minutes

The Total Preparation/Cook Time: 30 minutes

Number of Calories in Individual Servings: 152

Protein Grams: 15

Phosphorus Milligrams: 257

Potassium Milligrams: 419

Sodium Milligrams: 65

Fat Grams: 5

Total Carbohydrates Grams: 9

Net Carbohydrates Grams: 7

The Ingredients:

Chicken breast, cut into strips - .25 pound

Onion powder - .25 teaspoon

Black pepper, ground - .25 teaspoon

Dill, dried - .5 teaspoon

Parsley, dried – 1 teaspoon

Garlic powder - .25 teaspoon

Sesame seed oil - .5 teaspoon

Cucumber, thinly sliced – 1

Lettuce – 1 cup

Pita bread – 2

Hummus - .25 cup

The Instructions:

1. Preheat your oven to a temperature of Fahrenheit four-hundred degrees.

2. Place the chicken strips on a small baking sheet and toss them together with the onion powder, black pepper, dried dill, dried parsley, garlic powder, and sesame seed oil. Ensure that they are fully coated and then place it in the oven until the chicken strips are fully cooked. This should take twenty to twenty-five minutes. The

middle of the chicken must reach a minimum temperature of Fahrenheit one-hundred and sixty-five degrees.

3. Once the chicken is done cooking, remove it from the oven and prepare the remaining aspects of your sandwiches. You need to cut the pita bread in half and then open the pockets with your hands or a fork. Slice the cucumbers, and tear the lettuce into bite-sized pieces.

4. First fill the pita bread halves with the lettuce, then the cucumber, and lastly the cooked chicken strips. Serve it immediately to prevent the pita from going stale and while the chicken is still warm.

Chicken and Rice Soup

This soup is quick and easy to make, and perfect for a cold winter day or for whenever you are feeling under the weather. However, keep in mind that you should plan this soup for on a day that you have other low-potassium meals planned. This is because while this soup is still classified as low-potassium, it does contain a little more potassium than many of the other recipes in this book.

While you can use low-sodium chicken broth from the store, you are best off using completely homemade broth so that you can ensure it has no added sodium.

The Details:

The Number of Servings: 2

The Time Needed to Prepare: 5 minutes

The Time Required to Cook: 25 minutes

The Total Preparation/Cook Time: 25 minutes

Number of Calories in Individual Servings: 374

Protein Grams: 19

Phosphorus Milligrams: 248

Potassium Milligrams: 649

Sodium Milligrams: 122

Fat Grams: 9

Total Carbohydrates Grams: 51

Net Carbohydrates Grams: 48

The Ingredients:

Chicken broth, low-sodium – 1 cup

Water – 2 cups

Onion, dehydrated flakes – 1 tablespoon

Garlic, minced – 4 cloves

Celery, diced – 1 rib

Carrots, sliced – 2

Chicken breast, sliced into small cubes - .25 pound

White rice, raw - .5 cup

Poultry seasoning - .5 teaspoon

Black pepper, ground - .25 teaspoon

Olive oil – 1 tablespoon

The Instructions:

1. In a large pot add in the olive oil along with the garlic, celery, and carrots. Cook them over medium heat. Allow these to sauté together for five minutes and then add in the remaining ingredients. Stir the pot together well and bring it to a boil over medium-high heat.

2. Once the pot comes to a boil, reduce it to a simmer, cover it with a lid, and allow it to cook until the rice and chicken are cooked about twenty minutes.

3. Turn off the heat, allow the soup to sit for five minutes, and then serve.

Shepherd's Pie

This recipe is made with mashed cauliflower instead of potatoes, making it much lower in potassium than traditional Shepherd's pie. Not only that, but it is full of vegetables! In a single serving, you can get nearly half of your daily serving of vegetables.

The Details:

The Number of Servings: 2

The Time Needed to Prepare: 5 minutes

The Time Required to Cook: 35 minutes

The Total Preparation/Cook Time: 40 minutes

Number of Calories in Individual Servings: 210

Protein Grams: 14

Phosphorus Milligrams: 192

Potassium Milligrams: 632

Sodium Milligrams: 94

Fat Grams: 11

Total Carbohydrates Grams: 13

Net Carbohydrates Grams: 10

The Ingredients:

Cauliflower, florets – 2 cups

Turkey, ground - .25 pound

Carrots, diced – 1

Corn kernels - .25 cup

Celery, diced – stalk

Poultry seasoning – 1 teaspoon

Black pepper, ground - .25 teaspoon

Olive oil - .5 tablespoon

The Instructions:

1. Place the cauliflower in a microwave-safe bowl with some water and cover it with a plate, and then microwave it until fork-tender. You can also steam it on the stove in a steam basket if you wish.

2. While your cauliflower is steaming, allow the oven to preheat to a temperature of Fahrenheit four-hundred degrees.

3. In a large skillet sauté the carrots and celery in the olive oil for five minutes. Add in the ground turkey and brown it until there is no pink remaining, about nine minutes. Stir in the corn, half of the black pepper, and three-quarters of the poultry seasoning.

4. In a medium-sized kitchen bowl mash, the cauliflower with a hand-held potato masher until it is nice and creamy. Add in the remaining black

pepper and poultry seasoning. Set aside the mashed cauliflower.

5. Spread the meat and vegetable mixture into the bottom of a loaf pan. Spread the cauliflower evenly over the top, and then allow it to cook in the preheated oven for twenty minutes. If you want, the last two minutes you can turn the oven's broiler on to get the mashed cauliflower nice and golden.

Type 5/Dialysis

Eggs with Green Chilies

This flavorful egg casserole is the perfect way to get the extra protein needed when on dialysis. Enjoy this for an easy and delicious breakfast, or a no-fuss dinner.

The Details:

The Number of Servings: 2

The Time Needed to Prepare: 5 minutes

The Time Required to Cook: 20 minutes

The Total Preparation/Cook Time: 25 minutes

Number of Calories in Individual Servings: 259

Protein Grams: 24

Phosphorus Milligrams: 343

Potassium Milligrams: 384

Sodium Milligrams: 238

Fat Grams: 13

Total Carbohydrates Grams: 8

Net Carbohydrates Grams: 8

The Ingredients:

Egg whites – 1 cup

Whole eggs – 1

Cheddar cheese, shredded, low-sodium – .5 cup

All-purpose flour – 1 tablespoon

Black pepper, ground - .125 teaspoon

Parsley, dried – .5 teaspoon

Onion, diced - .25 cup

Garlic, minced – 2 cloves

Bell pepper, diced - .25 cup

Green chilled, canned, rinsed – 2 tablespoons

The Instructions:

1. Preheat your oven to a temperature of Fahrenheit three-hundred and fifty degrees and grease a regular-sized loaf pan for the egg casserole.

2. In a medium-sized bowl for the purpose of mixing whisk together the egg whites and whole egg until the two are completely combined. Whisk in the remaining ingredients.

3. Pour the prepared egg, vegetable, and cheese mixture into the greased loaf pan and then place

it in the center of the oven, allowing it to cook until it has set and the eggs are cooked all the way through, about twenty to twenty-five minutes.

Quinoa Breakfast Bowls

These quinoa breakfast bowls are packed with protein and flavor! You will love how the blueberries and cinnamon complement the seeds. This is a wonderful way to start your morning.

The Details:

The Number of Servings: 2

The Time Needed to Prepare: 5 minutes

The Time Required to Cook: 20 minutes

The Total Preparation/Cook Time: 25 minutes

Number of Calories in Individual Servings: 270

Protein Grams: 11

Phosphorus Milligrams: 256

Potassium Milligrams: 376

Sodium Milligrams: 86

Fat Grams: 6

Total Carbohydrates Grams: 44

Net Carbohydrates Grams: 40

The Ingredients:

Water - .5 cup

Tofu, silken - .5 cup

Almond milk - .75 cup

Quinoa, raw, rinsed well - .5 cup

Brown sugar – 1.5 tablespoons

Vanilla extract - .5 teaspoon

Cinnamon, ground - .25 teaspoon

Blueberries, fresh - .5 cup

The Instructions:

1. In a blender combine the silken tofu, water, and almond milk until smooth. This shouldn't take much work, as the tofu is really soft.

2. Once blended, pour the almond milk and tofu mixture into a large saucepan and add in the quinoa and vanilla extract. Allow this quinoa mixture to come to a boil over a temperature of medium-high heat. Be sure to stir the mixture occasionally.

3. Once the quinoa has reached a boil, reduce the heat to low and cover it with a lid, allowing it to simmer for fifteen minutes while continuing to stir occasionally.

4. Stir the brown sugar and cinnamon into the quinoa and then allow it to cook with the lid on for an additional five minutes, or until most of the liquid has been absorbed by the quinoa.

5. Serve the quinoa, topping it with the blueberries.

Italian Herb Chicken and Asparagus

This dish is full of healthy protein from chicken and low in saturated fats. You will love the way that the herbed chicken pairs with the fresh asparagus and mild white rice. Enjoy it for either a high-protein lunch or dinner.

The Details:

The Number of Servings: 2

The Time Needed to Prepare: 5 minutes

The Time Required to Cook: 15 minutes

The Total Preparation/Cook Time: 20 minutes

Number of Calories in Individual Servings: 331

Protein Grams: 22

Phosphorus Milligrams: 259

Potassium Milligrams: 475

Sodium Milligrams: 38

Fat Grams: 9

Total Carbohydrates Grams: 38

Net Carbohydrates Grams: 36

The Ingredients:

Chicken breast, cut into bite-sized pieces – .33 pound

Italian herb seasoning – 2 teaspoons

Black pepper, ground – .25 teaspoon

Lemon zest - .25 teaspoon

Garlic, minced – 3 cloves

Olive oil – 1 tablespoon

Asparagus, cut into bite-sized pieces - .33 pound

Rice, white, cooked – 1.5 cups

The Instructions:

1. Preheat your oven to a temperature of Fahrenheit four-hundred and fifty degrees before covering a large sheet pan with kitchen parchment.

2. In a small bowl toss together the chicken, asparagus, herb seasoning, black pepper, lemon zest, garlic, and olive oil. You want to ensure that all of the ingredients are evenly coated. Either cook this mixture right away or allow it to marinate for fifteen minutes.

3. Place the coated asparagus and chicken onto the baking pan and allow it to cook until the chicken reaches an internal temperature of Fahrenheit one-hundred and sixty-five degrees and the asparagus is tender about fifteen to twenty minutes.

4. Remove the pan from the oven and either immediately serve it over the rice, or store it in the fridge or freezer to enjoy at a later date.

Barbecue Tofu and Rice

This recipe makes faux-barbecue tofu. While barbecue sauce is not allowed on the kidney disease diet due to its high sodium and potassium contents, this recipe utilizes seasonings to make a similar barbecue flavor, but without the use of sodium or potassium-rich tomatoes. If you are a barbecue lover, you will absolutely love this tofu! Of course, you can also make it with chicken, if you wish.

This recipe makes use of onion powder and garlic powder, please keep in mind that these are very different from onion and garlic salt. Unlike the ladder, these do not contain added sodium and can be used on the kidney disease diet.

The Details:

The Number of Servings: 2

The Time Needed to Prepare: 5 minutes

The Time Required to Cook: 15 minutes

The Total Preparation/Cook Time: 20 minutes

Number of Calories in Individual Servings: 462

Protein Grams: 25

Phosphorus Milligrams: 368

Potassium Milligrams: 393

Sodium Milligrams: 23

Fat Grams: 20

Total Carbohydrates Grams: 46

Net Carbohydrates Grams: 44

The Ingredients:

Tofu, extra firm, cut into bite-sized cubes – 16 ounces

Corn starch – 1 tablespoon

Red wine vinegar – 2 tablespoons

Onion powder - .25 teaspoon

Brown sugar – 2 teaspoons

Smoked paprika - 1 teaspoon

Cayenne pepper - .125 teaspoon

Olive oil – 2 tablespoons

Garlic powder - .25 teaspoon

Black pepper, ground - .25 teaspoon

Rice, white, cooked - .1.5 cups

The Instructions:

- Heat a skillet over medium-high heat and add in the olive oil. While you can use a stainless-steel skillet, it is easier to use a non-stick skillet.

- In a medium-sized bowl add in the corn starch, cayenne pepper, onion powder, smoked paprika, garlic powder, black ground pepper, and brown sugar. Whisk these together and then add in the tofu, tossing them together until the tofu is fully coated. Add int eh red wine vinegar and toss the mixture together again.

- Place the tofu cubes in the hot oil of the skillet, giving them each a little space between the cubes so that they are not sticking. After a couple of minutes flip them over, and continue to do this until all sides of the cubes are golden in color. Remove the tofu from the skillet, and if you have any remaining uncooked cubes, cook them now, as well.

- Serve the barbecue tofu over the white rice and enjoy!

Conclusion

While you previously likely had very little knowledge about how your kidneys function, their ability to manage mineral and fluid levels in your body, how they synthesize vitamin D so that it's usable by for your cells, and, of course, how they produce urine through the process of removing toxins and waste from your blood. These organs might be little, but they are mighty. Sadly, over thirty million Americans mighty kidneys are being affected and degraded by chronic kidney disease, high blood pressure, and diabetes.

Thankfully, with the help of Dr. Robert Porter and Dr. Elizabeth Torres, you now have all the information you need to get well on your way to successfully treat your kidney disease! Through a healthy lifestyle and the kidney disease diet, you can halt the damage to your kidneys in its tracks, hopefully preventing the need for dialysis or transplantation in the future. Not only that, but you also learned about some amazing therapies that are now available and will be available in the future, which should give you hope.

If you found the knowledge and information imparted by Dr. Porter and the delicious and nutritious recipes shared by Dr. Torres helpful, then you should check out their other book. With **The Renal Diet Cookbook,** you will have access to even more recipes to make your life on the kidney disease diet easier. Along with many more recipes, you will also get helpful information on menu planning, so be sure to check it out!

Thank you for reading *the Kidney Disease Diet*. We hope that with the information you have learned, you will soon gain a healthier and happier lifestyle. You can enjoy gaining healthier kidneys, lower blood pressure, reduced cholesterol, and healthier blood sugar. By combining this book with a close relationship with your doctor, you can live better and longer.

Renal Diet Cookbook

An Easy-to-Follow Guide to Stop Kidney Disease with Healthy and Delicious Renal Diet Recipes

Part I

Introduction

The kidneys are two bean-shaped organs that we all know about in passing. However, they are still greatly underappreciated. While people may know that they are a set of two organs which are a part of the urinary tract, too few people appreciate and understand the vital importance of these organs. Not only do kidneys help in the production of urine, but they also filter waste and toxins from our blood, remove these particles from our bodies, manage fluid and mineral levels, and synthesize vitamin D so that it can be utilized by our cells. With all of the abilities of our kidneys, people are in a dangerous state when they have chronic kidney disease. Not only does this disease cause a person's kidney disease functioning to lessen, but it also can lead to kidney failure. When a person develops kidney failure, they are unable to survive without either transplantation or blood dialysis treatments multiple times a week.

Sadly, the number of cases of chronic kidney disease is only on the rise in the United States and other Western countries. With high blood pressure and diabetes also on the rise, which is both primary culprits for having kidney disease, the damage to peoples' kidneys is only worsening as time goes on. Without treating both kidney disease and the condition that predisposed a person for the disease, such as high blood pressure or diabetes, a person can not expect to get better.

Thankfully, there is an option. The chronic kidney disease diet does not only treat kidney disease, but it also treats both diabetes and high blood pressure allowing a person to frequently stop the spread of kidney damage. The purpose of this is to hopefully prevent kidney failure before it happens, and if a person does develop kidney failure, to then manage the condition along with other necessary treatments.

In Renal Diet Cookbook, Dr. Robert Porter will help you better understand kidney functioning and health while Dr. Elizabeth Porter provides you with over sixty recipes to enjoy on the kidney disease diet and lifestyle.

No longer do you have to simply accept the progression of chronic kidney disease. You can now use a healthy and delicious renal diet to increase the health of your kidneys and improve your entire life.

Chapter 1: Kidney Function 101

The kidneys are two incredibly powerful organs. When a person has two healthy and fully functioning kidneys, these organs can filter four ounces of blood removing waste and impurities from it every minute. During the process of filtering this blood, not only do the kidneys remove waste, but they also remove a little excess fluid to create urine and remove the waste. After this process, the waste-filled fluid is pushed to the bladder where it will become urine before being expelled from the body.

Since the kidneys filter the blood, people may mistakenly believe that the kidneys are like a sponge that absorbs and hold onto any waste or impurities. However, this is not true. The kidneys may remove waste and toxins from the blood, but rather than holding onto it, they have a process to eliminate it in our system.

The kidneys will also remove some excess acid from your blood, which is a production of your blood used to maintain healthy levels of water and minerals. This acid affects many minerals, but most notably phosphorus, potassium, sodium, and calcium. When these minerals become unbalanced, it leads to a host of problems, such as trouble balancing and an inability of the muscles, tissues, and nerves to function properly. This can become incredibly dangerous.

Since the kidneys cannot manage anymore the levels of acid in your blood or properly manage your mineral levels, it can lead to a dangerous buildup, which is just as damaging to your body as a deficit. For this reason, people with chronic kidney disease (CKD) have to manually manage their mineral intake to prevent buildup.

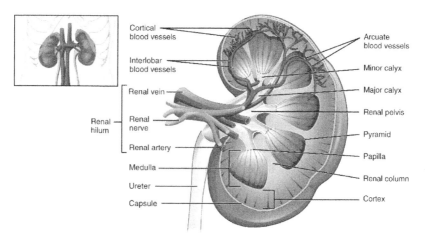

But, who is most at risk of chronic kidney disease? You might be reading this book if you have already been diagnosed, but you may also be reading it if your doctor suspects kidney disease or if a family member has been diagnosed. Therefore, it is important to understand the risk factors of the disease, so that you can better know if you or your loved ones are at risk.

Firstly, people with a family history of kidney disorders, high blood pressure, or diabetes have a higher chance of developing CKD. Although, there are also other people with an increased risk, which include the elderly, black people, Latinx people, Native people, and Pacific Islanders.

There are also many conditions that can directly cause chronic kidney disease. This includes kidney inflammation, high blood pressure, urinary tract infections, renal cancer, and type I and type II diabetes. In fact, renal cancer is one of the most common types of cancer in the United States, being the seventh most common. Two-thirds of the chronic kidney illnesses' cases are because of high blood pressure and diabetes, meaning that not only do people need to treat their kidney health directly, but also indirectly by treating these two conditions. If a person has high blood pressure or diabetes with kidney disease and doesn't treat the former, then these conditions will only worsen kidney health and potentially lead to kidney failure.

If you're at risk of having a disease in your kidneys have increased, your doctor suspects you might have already developed it, then they will likely run a series of tests. These frequently include blood pressure, serum creatinine, and urine albumin tests. If a person experiences increased markers on these three tests, they will likely receive a diagnosis for chronic kidney disease or another kidney condition. Testing for CKD is really simple and a quick process, allowing your doctor to run regular yearly tests if you are concerned about your kidney health due to increased risk of developing the disease.

While chronic kidney disease is one of the more common and dangerous kidney conditions, there are other conditions related to poor kidney health as well. The dangers of CKD is that it can easily cause dangerous side effects if a person doesn't eat well and it can develop into full-on kidney failure.

With chronic kidney disease, when left untreated, a person's kidneys slowly degrade and take on more damage as they decrease in their ability to function. If a person reaches kidney failure, they are in stage five of the disease which is the most severe. With this stage, a person is unable to survive unless they seek medical attention in the way of transplantation or blood dialysis treatment.

If are in need of a transplant down the road, you will be happy to know those healthy individuals can donate their kidneys. Not only can someone donate one of their whole kidneys, but they can also donate simply a portion of their kidneys to help someone who has reached kidney failure. Many people seek to donate their kidneys when a family member or friend is in need, however, it is also possible for people with healthy kidneys to donate their kidneys to strangers in need.

Thankfully, if someone is hoping to donate their kidney, they do not have to worry about its safety. Of course, there are always risks with any surgery no matter how minor. However, kidney removal and transplantation are one of the most common surgeries in the United States, meaning that there is less risk than many other surgeries. If a person is interested in donating an organ, they should contact their doctor who can discuss the risks, benefits, and walk them through the process.

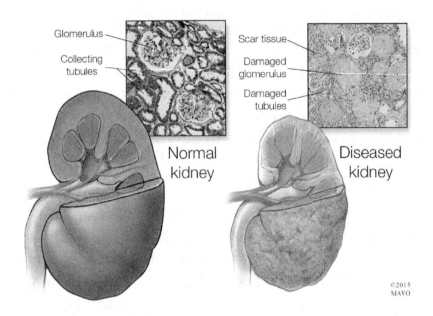

Glomerulus

Collecting tubules

Scar tissue

Damaged glomerulus

Damaged tubules

Normal kidney

Diseased kidney

©2015 MAYO

If you are diagnosed with chronic kidney disease, your doctor will use a test known as a glomerular filtration rate (GFR) to understand which stage of the disease you are in. By knowing what stage of the disease you are in, a doctor can better understand how damaged your kidneys are and how likely kidney failure is to develop. Not only that, but your treatment needs and dietary requirements change depending on what level of CKD you are in.

4. **Stage One**

A person has normal GFR results (≥ 90 mL/min/1.73 m2) along with persistent excessive albumin protein in the urine, structural kidney disease, or hereditary kidney disease. Kidney damage may also be viewable through an ultrasound, CT scan, X-ray with contrast, and an MRI.

- **Stage Two**
  GFR results 60 to 89 mL/min/1.73 m2. At this point, the person is unlikely to be experiencing symptoms from the disease. Therefore, if the disease is discovered this early, it is often only due to the treatment of another disease such as diabetes or high blood pressure.

- **Stage Three A.**
  GFR results 45 to 59 mL/min/1.73 m2. A person may start to experience symptoms during stage three (either type A. or B.). These may include fatigue, lower back pain, shortness of breath, swelling, fluid retention, urination changes, muscle cramps, restless legs, or trouble sleeping. These symptoms are the same in both types of stage three.

- **Stage Three B.**
  GFR results 30 to 44 mL/min/1.73 m2

- **Stage Four**
  GFR results 15 to 29 mL/min/1.73 m2. Along with the symptoms in stage three, a person may experience additional symptoms in stage four. These symptoms can include bad breath, taste changes, loss of appetite, vomiting, nausea, difficulty concentrating, and nerve problems such as numbness and tingling.

- **Stage Five**
  GFR results <15 mL/min/1.73 m2. Along with the symptoms of the previous stages, a person in stage five (kidney failure) may experience itching, skin color changes, puffy eyes, and

little to no urination.

When you have chronic kidney disease, the most important thing to remember is to always be careful about what you are putting in your body. This, of course, means fluids and foods, but it also includes what medications you take. For instance, many over-the-counter medications are not safe for those with decreased kidney health. Smoking will also decrease your risk.

However, while all lifestyle factors can impact kidney health, in this book, we will be focusing on how diet affects your kidney health and provide you with recipes to maintain a healthy and delicious kidney-friendly diet.

New and Exciting Therapies and Treatments for Chronic Kidney Disease

One common problem of chronic kidney disease is protein leakage from the kidneys. This is known as proteinuria. This problem is dangerous on its own, but it also further worsens kidney disease. Thankfully, there is a brand new and breakthrough drug therapy that can help decrease proteinuria and alleviate some of the damage that it causes. This is a wonderful answer which can decrease future kidney damage in people all around the world.

This new drug therapy uses what is known as a blocker compound, which is combined with another blocker compound frequently in the treatment of high blood pressure and nephropathy in people with type II diabetes. These two blockers are being used in conjunction, as researchers found that they beneficially interact with kidney cell receptors.

Nearly half of the people who have chronic kidney disease also have diabetes, which is startling. Thankfully, there is new hope for patients who have both type II diabetes and chronic kidney disease. In trials on new drug therapy, with the medicine canagliflozin, researchers found that the medication offered new options in reducing the production of the kidney disease. This is especially exciting, as it is the first time in more than fifteen years that success such as this has been reached.

This trial consisted of a large pool of individuals, which means that it is incredibly sound. Four-thousand and four-hundred individuals participated, finding that canagliflozin (sold under Invokana) can help stop the progression of the disease safely. In fact, the trial was able to end sooner than was originally planned, as it was proven to be safe and effective more quickly than researchers had hoped.

While there are some medications that lower blood pressure and reduce the risk of chronic kidney disease, these other medications are only partially effective. On the other hand, Invokana, a small daily pill meant to control blood sugar, has been shown to be much more effective in the reduction in the risk of kidney failure and prevention of chronic kidney disease. The study found that the participants on Invokana experienced a thirty percent lower chances of kidney failure, the requirement for dialysis treatment, required kidney transplantation, or death related to either kidney or heart problems.

Worldwide, there are one hundred and sixty million people with type II diabetes who have a higher chance of having chronic kidney disease. With this new medication option on the horizon, it offers new options in preventing the risk of kidney failure, transplantation, and dialysis. The importance of these results can not be overstated.

In the future, the need for kidney transplantation might decrease. While the demand for transplantation has only increased in recent years, as kidney disease, high blood pressure, and diabetes are on the rise, the future offers new hope. Why is this? It is all thanks to the ongoing research in stem cells and their ability to heal.

While patients won't see the results of stem cell research for years to come, scientists have found several exciting possibilities. For instance, researchers are currently studying how it is possible for the kidneys to regenerate themselves rather than requiring transplantation. To this end, researchers are attempting to discover which type of kidney cells are needed for the process.

As kidney disease is a result of different cell types being damaged in the kidneys, researchers must consider which cells are damaged. This means that stem cell treatments are only effective when researchers know which cells were damaged and need replacement.

While it is still yet to be clear which type of cells are needed for kidney regeneration, there are several groups of cells that are being investigated. Some of these cells that are located around the nephrons possess characteristics similar to stem cells. One of the cell groups currently being investigated is the renal progenitor cells. There is another type of cell that is also being investigated, which is similar to the cells found in bone marrow, known as mesenchymal stem cells.

One type of stem cell being used in ongoing research is the pluripotent stem cells. These cells are being used to create 3D structures similar to the nephrons of our kidneys. The purpose of this is to analyze how they are formed in embryos, test new drug therapy options, and create the possibility of replacing the nephrons on damaged kidneys in the future.

As you can see, there are some exciting new possibilities now available for those with chronic kidney disease, with more opportunities being researched for the future. We discuss more new therapies, treatments, and medications in our other book, *Kidney Disease Diet*.

Chapter 2: Meal Planning with Kidney Disease

In this chapter, we will explore how you can plan your diet while taking the best care of your kidneys as possible. We will look at not only how you should eat when you have chronic kidney disease, but how different stages of the disease can affect your diet.

Kidney Disease Diet for Stages One Though Four

On all stages of the kidney disease diet, you need to limit sodium, potassium, and phosphorus. However, for those who are not on dialysis between stages one and four, protein should also be limited. Overall, your diet should consist of as many fruits and vegetables as you can consume without going over your daily intake of potassium and phosphorus. You want to consume refined grains rather than whole grains, as they are lower in these minerals. The healthier fats, such as olive oil, should be used in place of typically unhealthy fats to improve heart-health and in the process of kidney health. Nuts, seeds, beans, and lentils can all be enjoyed for their health benefits, but only in moderation due to their high mineral content. And lastly, sugar should be avoided, with only small amounts of natural sweeteners (honey and maple) and in the place of sugar natural alternatives (stevia and sugar alcohols).

Protein is an important aspect of a person's diet as it wards off infections, repairs cellular damage, and prevents muscle wasting. However, protein intake should be closely monitored for a person with chronic kidney disease. For a person in stages one through four, they will most likely be recommended decreased protein consumption by their doctor. While most adults are recommended 0.8 grams of protein per kilogram of body weight, there is not one set recommendation for people with chronic kidney disease. Therefore, you should ask your doctor or renal dietitian about your needed protein daily intake.

For people with chronic kidney disease, it is important to limit protein intake due to the waste byproducts in the protein. For most people, this waste is no problem, as the kidneys can filter it from the body. However, the same is not true of people whose kidneys lack full function. This causes waste to buildup in the bloodstream, worsening kidney damage and increasing the progression of the disease. Thankfully, studies have shown that by limiting protein intake, a person can slow the progression of their disease.

Not all protein is created equal. Try to limit red meat, as this will worsen high blood pressure and heart disease, which is not only bad for your heart, but also for your kidneys. Plant-based proteins are the ideal protein source for chronic kidney disease, as studies have found that by favoring plant-based proteins, people can lessen the progression of their disease. There are multiple reasons for this, partially because animal-based proteins are lower in harmful saturated fats. However, it is also due to the phosphorus found in these foods. Both meat and plant-based proteins contain phosphorus, but it is more bioavailable in meat, meaning that your body absorbs in more. On the other hand, the phosphorus in plant-based proteins has a limited bioavailability, which means less of it is absorbed to affect your kidneys.

Of course, you have to limit many plant-based proteins, such as beans, due to their mineral content. But, when possible, try to consume plant-based proteins such as tofu, edamame, beans, lentils, grains, seeds, and nuts.

There are nine essential amino acids, which are the building blocks of protein. In animal-based products, you get all nine of these needed amino acids. However, many plant-based foods contain only a handful of amino acids. You have to consume a variety of foods to consume all your needed amino acids. Thankfully, there are some sources of complete protein in plant-based products, meaning they have all of these nine amino acids. These complete plant-based proteins are:

- Quinoa
- Buckwheat
- Chia seeds
- Tofu
- Beans paired with rice

While the specific amount of protein a person with chronic kidney disease should eat in a day will vary depending on their doctor's recommendation, a common recommendation is between fifty and sixty grams. Let's look at one way you can consume this amount of protein with a mixture of both plant-based and animal-based proteins:

- Quinoa, cooked - .5 cup

- Yogurt, low-fat - .5 cup

- Beans, cooked - .5 cup

- Chicken breast – 4 ounces

With these few sources of protein throughout your day, you can consume fifty-three grams of protein. These four protein sources, when combined together, also contain 176 milligrams of sodium, 707 milligrams of phosphorus, and 1090 milligrams of potassium.

It is vital for sodium to be limited, which is in much more than just salt. You also find sodium in cheeses, meats, broths, and more. The problem is that these cause high blood pressure and worsen kidney damage. In general, if a person has healthy blood pressure, they can consume between two-thousand and three-thousand milligrams of sodium daily. This means that highly-processed foods, lunch meats, many canned foods (those that are high in sodium), and pre-prepared meals should all be avoided.

Phosphorus easily builds up in the bloodstream, worsening kidney damage. Again, your doctor should recommend a specific daily amount of phosphorus for you in order to limit your intake. The specific amount of phosphorus you can eat will vary, but generally, when a person reaches the end-stage of the disease (stage 5), they are advised to consume no more than one-thousand milligrams daily.

Calcium may be limited, which is not generally difficult, as many foods that are high in calcium are also high in phosphorus, meaning you will already be avoiding them.

Lastly, it is important to limit potassium. While your doctor will recommend a specific daily intake of potassium, in general, people in stage one through four shouldn't consume more than two-thousand milligrams daily. Potassium is a mineral easy to consume, as it is found in high number in many natural and healthy foods. However, when you have kidney disease, your kidneys are no longer able to filter out excess potassium from your bloodstream, causing a dangerous buildup.

Therefore, you have to limit it to make up for the inability of your kidneys.

Kidney Disease Diet for Stage Five and Dialysis Patients

The fifth stage of kidney disease, when a person usually begins dialysis unless they receive a transplant, looks different than the diet for stages one through four. In this stage, you need to take more precautions. This generally means you have to watch your mineral intake even more carefully, increase protein intake, and decrease fluid intake. Your doctor will recommend a specific mineral intake based on your needs, so let's look at the fluids and protein in more detail.

Fluids:

Often times, people do not consume enough water. However, people who are undergoing dialysis can easily develop a fluid overload known as hypervolemia. This is dangerous, as it can cause excessive swelling and difficulty in breathing.

When a person experiences kidney failure and begins dialysis, their kidneys are no longer able to balance fluid levels. This can lead to hypervolemia, which is incredibly dangerous. This side effect is the same reason as to why people need to be even more hypervigilant in limiting their sodium intake because sodium will increase the body's fluid levels. Thankfully, by reducing sodium and fluid levels, you can limit this.

If you are worried you might have consumed too much sodium or fluids, watch for telltale symptoms of hypervolemia, such as shortness of breath, cramping, headaches, high blood pressure, bloating, swelling, increased heart rate, and heart palpitations.

The exact amount of fluids you can consume will vary from person to person. Your doctor and dialysis team can discuss with you how many ounces of fluids you can drink in a day, including water, coffee, tea, and broth. However, while there is not one set recommendation, oftentimes, people are recommended no more than thirty-two ounces daily.

Doctors frequently recommend using ice chips, frozen grapes, and sugar-free hard candies to control thirst levels when limiting liquid intake.

Protein:

In general, people are recommended to limit their protein intake in stages one through four of chronic kidney disease. However, when a person is on dialysis in stage five, they are recommended the opposite. Since the process of dialysis can better manage the waste in your bloodstream, patients are instructed to increase healthy sources of protein, as these can help a person increase their overall health.

When increasing your protein, it is important that you don't reach for red meats, as these are high in saturated fats that will worsen blood pressure and kidney damage. Instead, try to enjoy poultry, fish, seafood, eggs, and plant-based proteins. You can also consume certain dairy products, but only in moderation due to their sodium, phosphorus, and potassium contents.

Foods to Enjoy and Avoid for Stages 1-5:

The following is a list of foods that you should avoid and those that you can enjoy. However, it is important to remember that just because something isn't listed here doesn't mean you can't strictly consume it. The foods not listed are often somewhere in-between the avoid and enjoy lists, meaning that you can enjoy them, but only in small quantity. Keep in mind that you can't freely eat as much as you want from the enjoy list, as these foods still contain a certain amount of phosphorus and potassium, meaning you have to take their nutritional data in mind. The easiest way to keep track of what you are eating and ensure you aren't eating too much potassium or phosphorus is to track your food with an app. Many smartphone diet apps will track not only what you eat, but the nutritional data of what you are eating. This means that you can see the number of minerals you are consuming, ensuring you aren't eating too many foods high in these minerals.

Avoid:	Enjoy:
Avocados	Turkey
Dark-colored sodas	Chicken
Whole grains	Salt-free broth/stock
High-sodium canned products	Fish
	Pork
Bananas	Beef
Cantaloupe	Seafood
Honeydew	White bread
Kiwi	White rice
Mango	Couscous
Nectarines	Pasta
Papaya	Pearled barley
Milk (limit dairy in general)	Egg noodles
	Almond milk, unsweetened
Processed meats	Rice milk, unsweetened
Oranges	Soy milk, unsweetened
Olives	Rice milk, unsweetened
Pickles	Apples
Relish	Carrots
Potatoes	

Sweet Potatoes
Apricots
Tomatoes
Pre-made meals and highly processed foods
Dates
Dried fruits
Swiss chard
Spinach
Beet greens
Salty snack foods
Seasonings with salt
Chocolate drinks
Beer
Regular (non-Greek) yogurt
Oysters
Organ meat
Fish roe
Oat bran
Wheat bran
Brewer's yeast
Grapefruit juice
Pomegranate juice
Parsnips
Rutabagas
Tomatoes
Beets
Artichoke
Squash, both winter and summer
Okra
Parsnips
Table salt

Cucumbers
Grapes
Celery
Berries
Green beans
Corn
Radishes
Peach
Cherries
Pineapple
Cottage cheese
Parmesan cheese
Feta cheese
Blue cheese
Greek yogurt
Cream cheese
Neufchatel cheese
Apple juice
Cranberries
Watermelon
Plums
Pears
Asparagus
Kale
Eggplant
Cauliflower
Cabbage
Onions
Garlic
Herbs and spices (free of salt)
Peppers
Rhubarb
Mushrooms

Sea salt	Coffee (limited to 8 ounces
Garlic salt	Tea (limited to 16 ounces)
Seasoning salt	Beans and lentils (in moderation)
Soy sauce	
Onion salt	
Celery salt	
Meat tenderizer	
Lemon pepper.	
Oyster sauce	
Teriyaki sauce	
Barbecue sauce	
Cured foods, such as meats and vegetables	
Lunch meats	

Lifestyle Factors

Keep in mind that it is not only your diet that will affect your kidney health but also your other lifestyle factors. Exercise, sleep quality, alcohol intake, smoking, over the counter medications, and more can affect your kidney health. If you want to treat your chronic kidney disease, you don't only need to begin the kidney disease diet, but take it as a whole life approach, in which you improve various lifestyle factors as well. **How you can improve your lifestyle factors for better kidney health is further discussed in our other book, _Kidney Disease Diet_, also by Dr. Robert Porter and Dr. Elizabeth Torres.**

Part II

Note:

Pictures about medical recipes are Not included within this book.

Dr. Elizabeth Torres used her specialty (dietitian specialised in renal diet) to share recipes specifically for the kidney disease diet, complete with easy to follow
step-by-step instructions and nutritional information.

You will love these recipes, their ease, how they can benefit your health, and their flavor. These recipes are truly delicious, making the kidney disease diet enjoyable.

Chapter 3: Breakfast

In this chapter, you will find the perfect recipes to start out your morning! You will find low-protein options for stages 1-4 and high-protein options for those in stage 5 on dialysis.

Greek Yogurt Pancakes

These pancakes are quick and easy to whip up, perfect for any day of the week! Try topping them with sugar-free syrup or fresh fruit.

Chronic Kidney Disease Stage: 1-4

The Details:

The Number of Servings: 2

The Time Needed to Prepare: 2 minutes

The Time Required to Cook: 7 minutes

The Total Preparation/Cook Time: 9 minutes

Number of Calories In Individual Servings: 171

Protein Grams: 9

Phosphorus Milligrams: 217

Potassium Milligrams: 240

Sodium Milligrams: 56

Fat Grams: 6

Total Carbohydrates Grams: 19

Net Carbohydrates Grams: 19

The Ingredients:

- Eggs, large – 1
- Greek yogurt, low-fat - .25 cup
- Rice milk – 2 tablespoons
- Baking powder, low-sodium - .5 teaspoon
- All-purpose flour – 1/3 cup
- Olive oil - .5 tablespoon

The Instructions:

- Combine in a mixing dish the rice milk, Greek yogurt, and egg with a small whisk.

- Add the all-purpose flour and low-sodium baking powder to the bowl and whisk until everything is well combined. However, try to avoid mixing the pancake mixture too much; it is okay if there are small clumps.

- Heat an electric griddle or a skillet over medium to medium-high heat. Once hot, grease the skillet with the olive oil and pour the pancake batter into small circles on the pan.

- Allow the pancakes to cook until the dough is full of air bubbles and begins to look dry, then flip them over. Don't mess with the pancakes unless you are flipping them, as it can cause them to stick or break. Once the other side of the pancakes has become golden, remove them from the skillet and cook any leftover batter.

- Serve the pancakes immediately with your favorite toppings.

Cauliflower Breakfast Hash

This cauliflower hash makes a wonderful alternative to traditional potato hashes, which are too high in potassium to be allowed on the kidney diet. The spices and herbs will also increase the flavor, making this hash one of your favorites! Don't worry about the fat of the olive oil, as it is a source of heart-healthy fat.

Chronic Kidney Disease Stage: 1-4

The Details:

The Number of Servings: 2

The Time Needed to Prepare: 2 minutes

The Time Required to Cook: 10 minutes

The Total Preparation/Cook Time: 12 minutes

Number of Calories In Individual Servings: 277

Protein Grams: 7

Phosphorus Milligrams: 125

Potassium Milligrams: 304

Sodium Milligrams: 82

Fat Grams: 25

Total Carbohydrates Grams: 7

Net Carbohydrates Grams: 5

The Ingredients:

- Cauliflower florets – 1 cup
- Eggs – 2
- Onion, diced - .25 cup

- Bell pepper, diced - .25 cup
- Paprika – .5 teaspoon
- Cayenne pepper - .25 teaspoon
- Cilantro, dried – 1 teaspoon
- Cumin – .5 teaspoons
- Olive oil – 3 tablespoons

The Instructions:

5. In a small bowl, combine the paprika, cayenne pepper, dried cilantro, and cumin before setting the bowl of spices over to the side for later.

6. Place a large non-stick skillet on the stove over a temperature of medium heat. Add in the olive oil, diced bell pepper, diced onion, and cauliflower florets. Allow these vegetables to cook together until they become softened, about five minutes.

7. Sprinkle the prepared cumin and paprika spice mixture over the top of the vegetables and stir them together until completely combined. Place a lid over the skillet and continue to sauté the vegetables in the olive oil until the cauliflower is fork-tender. Occasionally remove the lid to stir the vegetables until they are ready.

8. Remove the lid from the skillet and make two "wells" in the vegetables big enough for the eggs. Crack one egg into each of the wells, cover the skillet with the lid again, and allow it to cook until the eggs are set. Remove away from the stove and serve within minutes.

Eggs with Green Chilies

This flavorful egg casserole is the perfect way to get the extra protein needed when on dialysis. Enjoy this for an easy and delicious breakfast or a no-fuss dinner.

Chronic Kidney Disease Stage: 5/Dialysis

The Details:

The Number of Servings: 2

The Time Needed to Prepare: 5 minutes

The Time Required to Cook: 20 minutes

The Total Preparation/Cook Time: 25 minutes

Number of Calories in Individual Servings: 259

Protein Grams: 24

Phosphorus Milligrams: 343

Potassium Milligrams: 384

Sodium Milligrams: 238

Fat Grams: 13

Total Carbohydrates Grams: 8

Net Carbohydrates Grams: 8

The Ingredients:

- Egg whites – 1 cup
- Whole eggs – 1
- Cheddar cheese, shredded, low-sodium – .5 cup
- All-purpose flour – 1 tablespoon

- Black pepper, ground - .125 teaspoon
- Parsley, dried – .5 teaspoon
- Onion, diced - .25 cup
- Garlic, minced – 2 cloves
- Bell pepper, diced - .25 cup
- Green chilled, canned, rinsed – 2 tablespoons

The Instructions:

9. Preheat your oven to a Fahrenheit temperature of three-hundred and fifty degrees and grease a regular-sized loaf pan for the egg casserole.

10.   In a medium-sized bowl for the purpose of mixing, whisk together the egg whites and whole egg until the two are completely combined. Whisk in the remaining ingredients.

11.   Pour the prepared egg, vegetable, and cheese mixture into the greased loaf pan and then place it in the center of the oven, allowing it to cook until it has set and the eggs are cooked all the way through, about twenty to twenty-five minutes.

Quinoa Breakfast Bowls

These quinoa breakfast bowls are packed with protein and flavor! You will love how the blueberries and cinnamon complement the seeds. This is a wonderful way to start your morning.

Chronic Kidney Disease Stage: 5/Dialysis

The Details:

The Number of Servings: 2

The Time Needed to Prepare: 5 minutes

The Time Required to Cook: 20 minutes

The Total Preparation/Cook Time: 25 minutes

Number of Calories In Individual Servings: 270

Protein Grams: 11

Phosphorus Milligrams: 256

Potassium Milligrams: 376

Sodium Milligrams: 86

Fat Grams: 6

Total Carbohydrates Grams: 44

Net Carbohydrates Grams: 40

The Ingredients:

- Water - .5 cup
- Tofu, silken - .5 cup
- Almond milk - .75 cup
- Quinoa, raw, rinsed well - .5 cup

- Brown sugar – 1.5 tablespoons

- Vanilla extract - .5 teaspoon

- Cinnamon, ground - .25 teaspoon

- Blueberries, fresh - .5 cup

The Instructions:

- In a blender, combine the silken tofu, water, and almond milk until smooth. This shouldn't take much work, as the tofu is really soft.

- Once blended, pour the almond milk and tofu mixture in a large casserole and add in the vanilla extract and quinoa. Allow this quinoa mixture to come to a boil over a temperature of medium-high heat. Be sure to stir the mixture occasionally.

- Once the quinoa boils, lower the heat's intensity and cover it with a lid, allowing it to simmer for fifteen minutes while continuing to stir occasionally.

- Stir the brown sugar and cinnamon into the quinoa and then allow it to cook with the lid on for an additional five mins or until the quinoa has almost absorbed all of the liquid.

- Serve the quinoa, topping it with the blueberries.

Maple Cinnamon French Toast

This delicious and simple French toast is a treat that can be enjoyed on all five stages of the kidney disease diet. However, it is important to remember that those in stages 1-4 require a low-protein diet, whereas it is important for those in stage 5 on dialysis to consume a higher protein content. Therefore, those in stage 5 should consider this meal with an added side of protein.

Chronic Kidney Disease Stage: 1-5/Dialysis

The Details:

The Number of Servings: 2

The Time Needed to Prepare: 5 minutes

The Time Required to Cook: 5 minutes

The Total Preparation/Cook Time: 10 minutes

Number of Calories In Individual Servings: 377

Protein Grams: 12

Phosphorus Milligrams: 178

Potassium Milligrams: 175

Sodium Milligrams: 244

Fat Grams: 15

Total Carbohydrates Grams: 43

Net Carbohydrates Grams: 42

The Ingredients:

- Rice milk – 1 cup

- Eggs – 3

- White bread, low-sodium, thickly cut – 4 slices

- Cinnamon - .25 teaspoon

- Olive oil – 1 tablespoon

- Maple syrup – 1 tablespoon

- Vanilla extract - .5 teaspoon

The Instructions:

- Set a large stewpot over a heat of medium temperature on the stove and add in the olive oil, allowing it to preheat while you quickly assemble the toast. It is best if the skillet is non-stick.

- In a dish of medium size, crack the eggs and then add in the rice milk, cinnamon, vanilla extract, and maple syrup. Use a whisk to combine a thick liquid, whisking until the egg whites are completely distributed.

- Once the mixture is done being whisked, add the bread, allowing it to soak for five to fifteen seconds before flipping it over and letting it soak for a few seconds again. The exact amount of time it soaks will depend on the density of the bread you use. You want it to soak long enough that the bread is completely soaked through, but not so long that it begins to fall apart.

- Add the toast to your skillet and allow the first side to cook until golden brown and it easily is removed from the pan. Don't try to flip it too soon, or else it will stick and fall apart. Once the first side is golden, about two minutes, flip it over and cook the other side for an additional two minutes.

- Serve the French toast immediately, either plain or with your favorite low-sugar topping.

Single-Serving Blueberry Muffin

This quick and simple single-serving blueberry muffin can be cooked in a mug and the microwave! Of course, if you would like to cook it in the oven, you can do so instead. For cooking this in the oven, simply set an oven or small toaster oven to a Fahrenheit temperature of three-hundred and fifty degrees and allow it to cook until fully set in the center, about twelve minutes.

If you intend to serve this muffin on stage 5/dialysis, you will need it with a side of added protein.

Chronic Kidney Disease Stage: 1-5/Dialysis

The Details:

The Number of Servings: 1

The Time Needed to Prepare: 2 minutes

The Time Required to Cook: 1.5 minutes

The Total Preparation/Cook Time: 3 minutes

Number of Calories In Individual Servings: 245

Protein Grams: 3

Phosphorus Milligrams: 127

Potassium Milligrams: 207

Sodium Milligrams: 25

Fat Grams: 7

Total Carbohydrates Grams: 41

Net Carbohydrates Grams: 40

The Ingredients:

- All-purpose flour - .25 cup
- Baking powder, low-sodium - .25 teaspoon
- Brown sugar – 1 tablespoon
- Olive oil – .5 tablespoons
- Cinnamon – pinch
- Almond milk – 2 tablespoons
- Blueberries – 1 tablespoon

The Instructions:

- Combine the low-sodium baking powder, brown sugar, all-purpose flour, and cinnamon together in a microwave-safe mug until the baking powder is fully combined into the other ingredients.

- Add the olive oil and almond milk to the mug and stir the ingredients together, just until incorporated. If needed, you can add an extra splash of almond milk. Fold in the blueberries, which can be either fresh or frozen.

- Place your mug of muffin dough in the microwave and allow it to heat on high for ninety seconds. Remove the muffin from the microwave and enjoy it either plain or with a slight drizzle of maple syrup.

Strawberry Scones

These scones are simple to make, but full of flavor and are fluffy! Perfect to enjoy on their own with a dab of butter or with a small amount of your favorite jam.

Chronic Kidney Disease Stage: 1-4

The Details:

The Number of Servings: 2

The Time Needed to Prepare: 5 minutes

The Time Required to Cook: 15 minutes

The Total Preparation/Cook Time: 20 minutes

Number of Calories In Individual Servings: 231

Protein Grams: 4

Phosphorus Milligrams: 127

Potassium Milligrams: 213

Sodium Milligrams: 25

Fat Grams: 10

Total Carbohydrates Grams: 29

Net Carbohydrates Grams: 28

The Ingredients:

- All-purpose flour - .5 cup
- Baking powder, low-sodium - .5 teaspoon
- Olive oil – 1.5 tablespoons
- Egg white – 1 tablespoon

- Almond milk – 2.5 tablespoons

- Sugar – 1 teaspoon

- Strawberries, sliced - .25 cup

The Instructions:

- Prepare a baking sheet by lining it with kitchen parchment and then set your oven to a Fahrenheit temperature of four-hundred degrees.

- In a small bowl for the purpose of mixing, combine the all-purpose flour and low-sodium baking powder. Once combined, mix in the olive oil until it forms a crumbly mixture. Add in the egg white, almond milk, and sugar.

- Once the batter is formed, gently fold the sliced strawberries into the scone mixture.

- Once the dough is formed, separate it into two portions, and then set these portions onto the prepared baking sheet. Form each of the two portions into a triangle or circle of even thickness and width. You want the scones to be about one to one and a half inches thick.

- Place the two prepared scones in the oven and allow them to bake until they just begin to turn slightly golden, and then remove them and allow them to cool for a few minutes. The scones should require about twelve to fifteen minutes in the oven.

Protein-Rich Vegetable Hash

This easy and simple hash is full of vegetables containing half of your daily vegetable needs. When possible, try to use high-quality roasted chicken that is organic and free of antibiotics, as high-quality protein will create less waste in your blood than cheaper protein sources.

Chronic Kidney Disease Stage: 5/Dialysis

The Details:

The Number of Servings: 1

The Time Needed to Prepare: 5 minutes

The Time Required to Cook: 15 minutes

The Total Preparation/Cook Time: 20 minutes

Number of Calories In Individual Servings: 356

Protein Grams: 31

Phosphorus Milligrams: 314

Potassium Milligrams: 439

Sodium Milligrams: 348

Fat Grams: 22

Total Carbohydrates Grams: 5

Net Carbohydrates Grams: 4

The Ingredients:

Radishes, quartered - .5 cup

Mushrooms, sliced - .25 cup

Bell pepper, diced - .25 cup

Chicken breast, roasted – 3 ounces

Feta cheese, crumbled – 1 ounce

Garlic powder - .25 teaspoon

Onion powder -.25 teaspoon

Olive oil – 1 tablespoon

The Instructions:

- Set your oven to a Fahrenheit temperature of four-hundred and fifty degrees and place the quartered radishes on a baking sheet. Allow these radishes to cook in the oven until they become fork-tender, about fifteen minutes.

- Once the radishes are done cooking, heat on the stove a large non-stick or cast iron pan with olive oil (one tablespoon) at a temperature of average heat.

- Add roasted radishes and remaining ingredients into the hot skillet and allow them to cook until deep golden brown. Every few minutes, stir the hash to allow it to cook on all sides, but be careful not to stir it too frequently. You want the hash to be able to sit in the skillet for a minute or two between stirring it, as this will allow the vegetables to sear.

- Once the hash has reached your preferred level of golden brown, remove it from the skillet and serve it immediately.

Fluffy Belgian Waffles

These Belgian waffles are perfectly fluffy and can be topped with practically anything. Whether you are in the mood for syrup, berries, compote, jam, or even savory toppings, you will find that these waffles are perfection.

If you are on stage five of chronic kidney disease and are on dialysis, keep in mind that these are low in protein and you will need to increase your protein content in your other meals or serve these waffles along with a side of protein.

Chronic Kidney Disease Stage: 1-5/Dialysis

The Details:

The Number of Servings: 1

The Time Needed to Prepare: 5 minutes

The Time Required to Cook: 10 minutes

The Total Preparation/Cook Time: 15 minutes

Number of Calories In Individual Servings: 279

Protein Grams: 6

Phosphorus Milligrams: 172

Potassium Milligrams: 224

Sodium Milligrams: 71

Fat Grams: 13

Total Carbohydrates Grams: 32

Net Carbohydrates Grams: 31

The Ingredients:

- Eggs – 1
- All-purpose flour, .5 cups, plus 1 tablespoon
- Baking powder, low-sodium - .5 teaspoon
- Olive oil – 1.5 tablespoons
- Almond milk - .5 cup
- Sugar - .75 teaspoon

The Instructions:

6. Before you begin to prepare your Belgian waffle batter, begin by preheating your waffle iron. You can use any waffle iron, although a Belgian waffle iron is ideal for fluffy and traditional waffles.

7. Mix in a bowl that is small in size the low-sodium baking powder, all-purpose flour, and sugar. Once combined, create a well in the middle of the mixture and break the egg into it. Combine the mixture lightly with a fork.

8. Add the almond milk and olive oil into the batter, and stir it together until moistened. There may be small clumps, which are okay, but you want to avoid an excessive number of clumps or overly large clumps.

9. Add the waffle batter into the waffle iron being careful to not overfill the iron. Cook the waffle until golden brown, remove it from the waffle iron and then cook the remaining batter.

10. Serve the waffles with your favorite toppings while still fresh and warm.

Chapter 4: Snack and Appetizers

These snacks and appetizers are the perfect way to lift your energy and keep you full all through the afternoon, to increase your appetite before a meal, or to serve at a party with all of your friends. Enjoy these snacks and appetizers whenever you find yourself needing a boost and you are sure to feel better.

Just remember, calculate the phosphorus, potassium, and sodium in these snacks into your daily goal, so that you don't absentmindedly consume too much.

Roasted Edamame

This edamame is the perfect way to lift your energy during the mid-afternoon, as it is a good low to moderate protein snack with heart-healthy olive oil.

Chronic Kidney Disease Stage: 1-5/Dialysis

The Details:

The Number of Servings: 2

The Time Needed to Prepare: 5 minutes

The Time Required to Cook: 15 minutes

The Total Preparation/Cook Time: 20 minutes

Number of Calories In Individual Servings: 279

Protein Grams: 8

Phosphorus Milligrams: 137

Potassium Milligrams: 357

Sodium Milligrams: 6

Fat Grams: 10

Total Carbohydrates Grams: 8

Net Carbohydrates Grams: 4

The Ingredients:

- Edamame, frozen, shelled – 1 cup
- Olive oil – 1 tablespoon
- Black pepper, ground - .25 teaspoon
- Garlic powder - .5 teaspoon
- Onion powder - .5 teaspoon

The Instructions:

5. Preheat your oven by setting it to a Fahrenheit temperature of four-hundred degrees and use a parchment paper in lining a baking sheet.

6. In a bowl, use a towel and dry the edamame until you have gotten all of the liquid off of them. Add in the olive oil and seasonings, tossing the edamame in them until they are completely and evenly coated. Spread the edamame on the prepared pan with kitchen parchment.

7. Place the edamame in the oven and allow it to roast until crispy, about fifteen to eighteen minutes.

Vanilla Frozen Blueberries

These frozen blueberries are coated in yogurt and lemon juice, giving them a sweet, creamy, and tangy taste. Perfect for a warm summer day, you will absolutely love these blueberries!

Chronic Kidney Disease Stage: 1-5/Dialysis

The Details:

The Number of Servings: 2

The Time Needed to Prepare: 10 minutes

The Time Required to Freeze: 2 hours

The Total Preparation/Cook Time: 130 minutes

Number of Calories In Individual Servings: 91

Protein Grams: 3

Phosphorus Milligrams: 86

Potassium Milligrams: 184

Sodium Milligrams: 38

Fat Grams: 1

Total Carbohydrates Grams: 18

Net Carbohydrates Grams: 17

The Ingredients:

- Blueberries – 1 cup
- Lemon juice – 1 teaspoon
- Vanilla yogurt, low-fat – 4 ounces

The Instructions:

4. Ensure that your blueberries are washed and dry, and then toss them in a bowl along with the lemon juice and yogurt. While doing this, be very gentle as you don't want the blueberries to become squished.

5. One by one, use a spoon or your hands to scoop out each blueberry, setting it on a baking sheet lined with kitchen parchment or wax paper. Ensure that the blueberries are not touching each other on the pan.

6. Place the baking sheet in the freezer and allow them to freeze for two hours. Remove the blueberries from the pan, setting them in either a plastic bag or container and store them in the freezer until you are ready to enjoy.

Cream Cheese Rangoon Rolls

These cream cheese rangoons are the perfect appetizer for any party. However, they are also so easy and quick to make that you can enjoy them any day of the week. Enjoy these alone or paired with your favorite low-sodium dipping sauce.

Chronic Kidney Disease Stage: 1-5/Dialysis

The Details:

The Number of Servings: 2

The Time Needed to Prepare: 5 minutes

The Time Required to Cook: 15 minutes

The Total Preparation/Cook Time: 20 minutes

Number of Calories In Individual Servings: 324

Protein Grams: 8

Phosphorus Milligrams: 83

Potassium Milligrams: 99

Sodium Milligrams: 470

Fat Grams: 15

Total Carbohydrates Grams: 38

Net Carbohydrates Grams: 37

The Ingredients:

- Egg roll wrappers – 4
- Cream cheese, softened – 2 ounces
- Garlic powder - .125 teaspoon

- Olive oil – 2 teaspoons
- Green onions, finely chopped – 1 tablespoon

The Instructions:

6. Prepare a baking sheet by coating it in kitchen parchment and preheat your oven to a Fahrenheit temperature of three-hundred and seventy-five degrees.

7. In a small-scaled dish, put together the green onions with the garlic powder and softened cream cheese.

8. In a small dish, add a small amount of water that you can dip your fingers in, and in another small dish, add your olive oil.

9. Lay out the four egg roll wrappers and divide the prepared cream cheese mixture between them. Place the cream cheese mixture on the bottom edge of the egg roll wrapper, keeping in mind it will expand as it cooks, so it's okay if it doesn't reach all the edges.

10. Dip your fingers in the prepared dish of water and then run your fingers along the top of the egg roll wrap, on the opposite side from the cream cheese. Ensure that you generously moisten the wrap.

11. Tightly wrap the egg roll wrap around the cream cheese, allowing the water to tightly seal it shut. If needed, you can add more water.

12. After the egg rolls are all tightly wrapped, place them on the prepared baking sheet and allow

them to cook for twelve to fifteen minutes until they are golden brown. You should flip them over halfway through the cooking process to ensure they cook evenly.

13. Serve the rolls alone or serve them alongside a kidney diet-friendly sauce that is low in sodium, phosphorus, and potassium.

Crispy Chocolate Clusters

No longer do you have to wish for sugar-laden chocolate bars. Instead, you can enjoy these homemade crispy rice and chocolate clusters. These use coconut oil, which is higher in saturated fat than olive oil, although it is a healthier type of saturated fat than what is found in animal-based products. In fact, coconut oil has been found to have many heart-healthy benefits. You can not replace the coconut oil with another, as coconut oil sets up firm when chilled, whereas many other oils do not.

Chronic Kidney Disease Stage: 1-5/Dialysis

The Details:

The Number of Servings: 2

The Time Needed to Prepare: 5 minutes

The Time Required to Cook: 15 minutes

The Total Preparation/Cook Time: 20 minutes

Number of Calories In Individual Servings: 114

Protein Grams: 8

Phosphorus Milligrams: 13

Potassium Milligrams: 64

Sodium Milligrams: 1

Fat Grams: 9

Total Carbohydrates Grams: 8

Net Carbohydrates Grams: 8

The Ingredients:

- Puffed white rice, plain - .25 cup
- Cocoa – 2 teaspoons
- Vanilla extract – .125 teaspoon
- Maple syrup – 2 teaspoons
- Coconut oil, melted – 4 teaspoons

The Instructions:

5. Together, in a small kitchen bowl, whisk the cocoa powder, vanilla extract, maple syrup, and melted coconut oil. Once it is completely smooth without any clumps, fold in the puffed white rice.

6. Use either a wax or parchment paper in lining a baking sheet. Then, use a spoon and create four mounds of the chocolate rice mixture on the baking sheet.

7. Place the baking sheet in the freezer for an hour until the mounds are flat. Remove them from the baking sheet and then store them either in a plastic bag or container until you are ready to enjoy.

Creamy Stuffed Celery

These celery boats are a much more fun and delicious version than your childhood snack of peanut butter and celery. You will love how the cream cheese and cheddar perfectly accent the celery.

Keep in mind that this recipe uses garlic powder, which is different from garlic salt. Don't ever use garlic salt on the kidney disease diet, as it is high in sodium.

Chronic Kidney Disease Stage: 1-5/Dialysis

The Details:

The Number of Servings: 2

The Time Needed to Prepare: 5 minutes

The Time Required to Cook: 0 minutes

The Total Preparation/Cook Time: 5 minutes

Number of Calories In Individual Servings: 255

Protein Grams: 6

Phosphorus Milligrams: 177

Potassium Milligrams: 219

Sodium Milligrams: 241

Fat Grams: 23

Total Carbohydrates Grams: 4

Net Carbohydrates Grams: 4

The Ingredients:

- Celery stalks, washed and dried – 2
- Cream cheese, softened – 4 ounces
- Cheddar cheese, low-sodium, grated - .25 cup
- Parsley, fresh, chopped – 2 teaspoons
- Chives, chopped – 2 teaspoons
- Black pepper, ground - .125 teaspoon
- Garlic powder - .125 teaspoon

The Instructions:

6. Slice your celery sticks into thirds or quarters, and then set them aside.

7. In a small bowl for the purpose of mixing, add the cream cheese, cheddar cheese, parsley, chives, black pepper, and garlic powder. Using a hand-held kitchen beater, whip the cream cheese mixture so that it is smooth and creamy.

8. Using a small spoon, fill the celery sticks with the cream cheese mixture and then serve immediately or store in the fridge and enjoy later in the afternoon.

Tuna Cucumber Bites

These tuna bites are the perfect way to increase your protein intake. Not only that, but they are delicious and easy to make!

Chronic Kidney Disease Stage: 5/Dialysis

The Details:

The Number of Servings: 2

The Time Needed to Prepare: 5 minutes

The Time Required to Cook: 0 minutes

The Total Preparation/Cook Time: 5 minutes

Number of Calories In Individual Servings: 118

Protein Grams: 19

Phosphorus Milligrams: 181

Potassium Milligrams: 370

Sodium Milligrams: 210

Fat Grams: 2

Total Carbohydrates Grams: 5

Net Carbohydrates Grams: 4

The Ingredients:

Tuna, light, canned – 1 can

Tofu, soft - .33 cup

Onion, thinly sliced - .33 cup

Cucumber, sliced – 1

Black pepper, ground - .25 teaspoon

Garlic powder - .25 teaspoon

The Instructions:

7. Place the black pepper, powder, and soft tofu garlic together in a bowl and then mash them together with a fork until the tofu is broken down.

8. Drain the light tuna and then add it to the tofu mixture along with the thinly sliced onion, and stir the mixture together until it is fully combined.

9. Slice your cucumber and then place the slices on a plate and top the slices off with the tuna mixture. Serve the tuna slices immediately.

Peanut Butter Yogurt

Enjoy this creamy and delicious yogurt either on its own or with a kidney disease diet-friendly fruit or cracker. Celery is even a good option!

Chronic Kidney Disease Stage: 5/Dialysis

The Details:

The Number of Servings: 2

The Time Needed to Prepare: 5 minutes

The Time Required to Cook: 0 minutes

The Total Preparation/Cook Time: 5 minutes

Number of Calories In Individual Servings: 264

Protein Grams: 15

Phosphorus Milligrams: 199

Potassium Milligrams: 346

Sodium Milligrams: 31

Fat Grams: 16

Total Carbohydrates Grams: 18

Net Carbohydrates Grams: 16

The Ingredients:

- Plain Greek yogurt - .5 cup
- Creamy peanut butter, low-sodium/no salt - .25 cup
- Honey – 1 tablespoon

The Instructions:

- Using a whisk, combine together the plain Greek yogurt, creamy peanut butter, and honey until it is smooth and without clumps. Serve it immediately or save it in the fridge to enjoy at a later date.

Parmesan Roasted Cauliflower

This roasted cauliflower is simple but absolutely delicious! Enjoy it served alone, or you can dip it in a low-sodium homemade mayonnaise made with olive oil.

Chronic Kidney Disease Stage: 1-5/Dialysis

The Details:

The Number of Servings: 2

The Time Needed to Prepare: 5 minutes

The Time Required to Cook: 20 minutes

The Total Preparation/Cook Time: 25 minutes

Number of Calories In Individual Servings: 144

Protein Grams: 5

Phosphorus Milligrams: 131

Potassium Milligrams: 360

Sodium Milligrams: 259

Fat Grams: 10

Total Carbohydrates Grams: 8

Net Carbohydrates Grams: 6

The Ingredients:

- Cauliflower florets – 2 cups
- Olive oil – 1 tablespoon
- Garlic powder - .5 teaspoon

- Black pepper, ground - .125 teaspoon

- Onion powder - .5 teaspoon

- Parmesan cheese, grated - .25 cup

The Instructions:

5. Preheat your oven to a temperature of four-hundred degrees Fahrenheit and then coat a cooking sheet with kitchen parchment.

6. In a mixing pot, blend together the grated Parmesan, onion powder, black pepper, garlic powder, olive oil, and cauliflower florets. Once the cauliflower is fully coated, transfer it to the prepared baking sheet.

7. Roast the cauliflower until golden brown and tender (20 mins). Remove the sheet from the oven and enjoy it immediately while still warm.

Crispy Kale Chips

These kale chips are quick and easy to cook, and they are incredibly healthy! If you want a small snack, but don't want to add to many added minerals or protein to your daily diet, then you can easily enjoy these and only increase your mineral content by a small amount. These are the perfect snack to enjoy when you are watching a movie and want a savory treat in place of popcorn.

Chronic Kidney Disease Stage: 1-5/Dialysis

The Details:

The Number of Servings: 2

The Time Needed to Prepare: 5 minutes

The Time Required to Cook: 20 minutes

The Total Preparation/Cook Time: 25 minutes

Number of Calories In Individual Servings: 130

Protein Grams: 0

Phosphorus Milligrams: 19

Potassium Milligrams: 97

Sodium Milligrams: 8

Fat Grams: 13

Total Carbohydrates Grams: 2

Net Carbohydrates Grams: 2

The Ingredients:

- Kale, chopped – 2 cups
- Olive oil – 2 tablespoons

- Onion powder - -25 teaspoon

- Onion powder - .25 teaspoon

- Parsley, dried - .5 teaspoon

- Dill weed, dried - .5 teaspoon

- Chives, dried - .5 teaspoon

The Instructions:

4. Preheat your oven to a Fahrenheit temperature of two-hundred and seventy-five degrees and then use a kitchen parchment when lining a baking pan.

5. Wash the kale leaves, ensure that they are dried completely, and then cut them into bite-sized pieces. Keep in mind that the leaves will shrink a small amount while they cook.

6. Place the kale in a large kitchen casserole and then blend them with the olive oil and seasoning until they are fully and evenly coated.

7. Lay the seasoned kale leaves out on the prepared cooking sheet in a single layer so that they do not overlap. This is important, as it ensures that the leaves cook evenly and become crispy.

8. Allow the kale to cook for ten minutes before flipping the leaves over and cooking an additional ten minutes until golden and crispy.

9. Serve the kale leaves immediately while hot, or let them cool and then store them in a plastic container to enjoy later on.

Chocolate Strawberry Bites

One of the great things about these strawberry bites is that you don't have to sit down and eat a full serving. While you can certainly enjoy a full serving if you only want one or two bites of sweetness, that's all you have to grab out of the freezer, as they can be stored ready and waiting for you to enjoy. Whether you have just gotten off of work or finished cleaning the kitchen, you can easily enjoy just one or two of these bites for a sweet treat without adding too many extra minerals to your daily diet.

Chronic Kidney Disease Stage: 1-5/Dialysis

The Details:

The Number of Servings: 2

The Time Needed to Prepare: 10 minutes

The Time Required to Freeze: 60 minutes

The Total Preparation/Cook Time: 70 minutes

Number of Calories In Individual Servings: 396

Protein Grams: 4

Phosphorus Milligrams: 188

Potassium Milligrams: 492

Sodium Milligrams: 12

Fat Grams: 28

Total Carbohydrates Grams: 30

Net Carbohydrates Grams: 23

The Ingredients:

- Strawberries, fresh - .25 pound

- Dark chocolate chips – 4 ounces

- Coconut oil – 2 teaspoons

The Instructions:

7. Slice the strawberries into quarters if they are large or in half if they are small. You want them in small bite-size pieces. Get a baking sheet ready with a wax or parchment paper.

8. In a microwave-safe bowl, add the dark chocolate chips and coconut oil, and then melt them in the microwave. In order to do this, microwave the chocolate for thirty seconds at a time, stirring it at the end of each thirty seconds until the chocolate is fully melted. Don't microwave them for longer periods without stirring, or else, the chocolate might burn.

9. Using a toothpick, pick up each strawberry piece and dip it in the chocolate mixture allowing it to become fully coated. Place the strawberry pieces on the prepared baking sheet when they are coated in chocolate

10. Place the strawberries in the freezer and allow them to chill until fully frozen, at least an hour. Once the chocolate is hardened, remove the frozen strawberries from the pan and put them in a container to be stored in the freezer until serving.

Cinnamon Candied Almonds

These almonds are full of flavor and much healthier than their sugary alternative! These use Truvia sweetener, which is a combination of sugar alcohol and stevia herb, which has been found safe in patients with kidney disease. The benefit of this is that unlike sugar, these will not worsen high blood sugar. Almonds are also a wonderful source of healthy fats and fiber, making them a known superfood.

Chronic Kidney Disease Stage: 1-5/Dialysis

The Details:

The Number of Servings: 2

The Time Needed to Prepare: 2 minutes

The Time Required to Cook: 7 minutes

The Total Preparation/Cook Time: 9 minutes

Number of Calories In Individual Servings: 212

Protein Grams: 7

Phosphorus Milligrams: 173

Potassium Milligrams: 268

Sodium Milligrams: 1

Fat Grams: 17

Total Carbohydrates Grams: 8

Net Carbohydrates Grams: 3

The Ingredients:

- Truvia sweetener – .25 cup

- Almonds, raw – .5 cup

- Cinnamon – 1 teaspoon

- Water – 1 tablespoon

- Vanilla extract - .25 teaspoon

The Instructions:

6. Place a skillet over medium heat and allow it to warm up. Once the skillet is hot, add in the Truvia sweetener, water, cinnamon, and vanilla extract. Using a spoon, combine the mixture and continue to stir it while it melts.

7. Once the Truvia mixture has completely melted, add in the almonds and stir to coat the almonds completely. Continue to stir and cook until the mixture begins to crystallize to the almonds, and then remove it from the heat.

8. Allow the almonds to sit for two to three minutes, and then use a spatula to break them apart before they stick together.

9. Allow the almonds to cool before serving them.

Chapter 5: Lunch

These lunches are perfect complete meals to enjoy in the afternoon, whether you are at home, the office, or on the road. You will be happy to know that these dishes are incredibly simple and easy to cook and are balanced meals.

Chicken Fajita Bowls

This meal is a perfect balance of meat, vegetables, and grains making it a great option to enjoy for lunch or dinner. You can easily serve this meal immediately or make it ahead of time and save it in the fridge to take with you to work for lunch.

Chronic Kidney Disease Stage: 1-4

The Details:

The Number of Servings: 2

The Time Needed to Prepare: 5 minutes

The Time Required to Cook: 15 minutes

The Total Preparation/Cook Time: 20 minutes

Number of Calories In Individual Servings: 365

Protein Grams: 17

Phosphorus Milligrams: 229

Potassium Milligrams: 510

Sodium Milligrams: 46

Fat Grams: 11

Total Carbohydrates Grams: 47

Net Carbohydrates Grams: 45

The Ingredients:

- Chicken breast - .25 pound
- Olive oil – 1.5 tablespoons
- Onion – 1
- Bell pepper, green – 1
- Bell pepper, red – 1
- Garlic, minced – 4 cloves
- Chili powder - .25 teaspoon
- Cayenne pepper – pinch
- Paprika - .25 teaspoon
- Cumin - .25 teaspoon
- Black pepper, ground - .25 teaspoon
- White rice, cooked – 1.5 cups

The Instructions:

- Combine the chili powder, cayenne pepper, paprika, cumin, and black pepper together to make your fajita seasonings and then set the spices aside.

- Slice the chicken breast into bite-sized cubes and then place it in a small bowl, massaging it with half of the prepared seasoning mix. Allow it to marinate for fifteen minutes.

- In a large-sized cooking pan warmed in a stove heat of medium with one tbps of the olive oil, cook the bell pepper and onion until soft, about five mins.

- Add in the chicken and garlic, and continue to cook until the chicken is fully cooked through, reaching an internal Fahrenheit temperature of one-hundred and sixty-five degrees. This should take about ten minutes. Don't forget to stir the chicken occasionally.

- The skillet should then be removed away from the stove's heat. Serve the vegetables and chicken over the rice.

Single Pan Balsamic Chicken and Veggies

This chicken and vegetable recipe is incredibly simple and only requires one pan! You can enjoy it either immediately for a fresh dinner or save it in the fridge or freezer for an easy lunch during the week.

Chronic Kidney Disease Stage: 1-4

The Details:

The Number of Servings: 2

The Time Needed to Prepare: 5 minutes

The Time Required to Cook: 15 minutes

The Total Preparation/Cook Time: 20 minutes

Number of Calories In Individual Servings: 346

Protein Grams: 18

Phosphorus Milligrams: 208

Potassium Milligrams: 504

Sodium Milligrams: 89

Fat Grams: 8

Total Carbohydrates Grams: 48

Net Carbohydrates Grams: 45

The Ingredients:

- Chicken, breast, cut into bite-sized pieces - .33 pound
- Baby carrots – 1 cup

- Onion, sliced – 1

- Italian herb seasoning – 1 teaspoon

- Balsamic vinegar – 1 tablespoon

- Olive oil – 1 tablespoon

- Black pepper, ground - .25 teaspoon

- Garlic, minced – 4 cloves

- Rice, white, cooked – 1.5 cups

The Instructions:

10. Preheat your oven to a Fahrenheit temperature of four-hundred degrees before lining a parchment paper in the tray for baking.

11. In a small bowl, use a whisk to combine together the olive oil, balsamic vinegar, Italian herb seasoning, black pepper, and minced garlic.

12. Place the bite-sized chicken pieces in a bowl and add in half of the vinegar and seasoning mix, massaging the mixture into the chicken. Allow the chicken to marinate for fifteen to thirty minutes ideally or use it right away.

13. Place the chicken and vegetables on the pan and toss them in the remaining prepared seasoning and vinegar mixture until evenly coated. Spread the vegetables and chicken out on the pan so that they cook evenly, and then set the pan into the center of your preheated oven.

14. Cook the mixture for fifteen minutes before turning the pan around to allow for even cooking, and then continue to cook for an additional fifteen minutes. Check and make sure that the chicken has reached an internal Fahrenheit temperature of one-hundred and sixty-five degrees. Remove the pan from the oven if it is ready, and if not, allow it to cook for a few more minutes.

15. Serve the vegetables and chicken over rice, either immediately or save them for lunch later in the week.

Pink Salmon with Roasted Broccoli

This salmon and roasted broccoli are delicious and extremely easy! Just keep in mind that the salmon is higher in potassium than poultry. However, as long as you make sure that the meals you eat during the remainder of your day don't put you over your potassium goal, then you should be okay. It is a good thing to include healthy fatty fish, such as salmon, which you can, as it has many health benefits and vital omega-3 fatty acids.

Chronic Kidney Disease Stage: 1-4

The Details:

The Number of Servings: 2

The Time Needed to Prepare: 5 minutes

The Time Required to Cook: 15 minutes

The Total Preparation/Cook Time: 20 minutes

Number of Calories In Individual Servings: 318

Protein Grams: 21

Phosphorus Milligrams: 301

Potassium Milligrams: 515

Sodium Milligrams: 81

Fat Grams: 11

Total Carbohydrates Grams: 32

Net Carbohydrates Grams: 31

The Ingredients:

- Salmon fillets – 6 ounces
- Cumin - .25 teaspoon
- Broccoli florets – 1 cup
- Olive oil – 1 tablespoon
- Lemon zest - .25 teaspoon
- Lemon juice – 2 teaspoons
- Garlic, minced – 2 cloves
- Red pepper flakes - .125 teaspoon
- Thyme, dried - .25 teaspoon
- Rice, white, cooked – 1.25 cups

The Instructions:

- Preheat your oven to a Fahrenheit temperature of four-hundred and twenty-five degrees and line a baking pan with kitchen parchment.

- In a baking sheet, lay down the broccoli florets, add the olive oil over the top, and toss the florets in the oil until they are evenly coated. Spread the florets around the pan.

- Set the salmon fillets on the baking pan between the broccoli florets.

- In a small bowl, combine the lemon zest, cumin, lemon juice, garlic, red pepper flakes, and thyme. Spread this mixture over the top of the salmon. Set the pan in the oven and allow it to cook until the salmon is cooked through and flaky, about ten to fifteen minutes.

- Withdraw from the oven the baking sheet and serve the rice, vegetables, and fish together. You may want to give a squeeze of fresh lemon over the top of it. It is also nice to add a little extra dried thyme and black pepper to the cooked rice.

Easy and Gourmet Pasta Salad

This pasta salad is full of nutrition, with homemade turkey meatballs, fresh mushrooms and asparagus, and heart-healthy olive oil. Enjoy this dish either immediately after making it, or enjoy it later on as a cold refrigerated treat.

Chronic Kidney Disease Stage: 1-4

The Details:

The Number of Servings: 2

The Time Needed to Prepare: 5 minutes

The Time Required to Cook: 20 minutes

The Total Preparation/Cook Time: 25 minutes

Number of Calories In Individual Servings: 474

Protein Grams: 22

Phosphorus Milligrams: 257

Potassium Milligrams: 419

Sodium Milligrams: 65

Fat Grams: 11

Total Carbohydrates Grams: 52

Net Carbohydrates Grams: 48

The Ingredients:

- Pasta, cooked – 2 cups
- Turkey, ground - .25 pound
- Italian seasoning – 1 teaspoon

- Bread crumbs, plain without seasonings – 1 tablespoon

- Black pepper, ground - .25 teaspoon

- Garlic minced – 3 cloves

- Mushrooms, sliced – .5 cup

- Asparagus - .25 pound

- Olive oil – 2 tablespoons

- Balsamic vinegar – 1 tablespoon

The Instructions:

- Start boiling a pot of water and let the pasta cook as per instructions. Meanwhile, preheat a saucepan of large size over a stove's medium heat temperature. Preferably, you want to use a non-stick skillet.

- While the skillet preheats, combine the ground turkey with the breadcrumbs, black pepper, minced garlic, and half of the Italian seasoning. Be careful not to over mix the meat, otherwise, it will become tough.

- Using a spoon, scoop out easily-sized portions and then roll them between your hands to form balls. You want each meatball to contain about two to three teaspoons of meat. Just be sure you don't heap the meat over the edge of the tablespoon, or else you will have too much meat mixture.

- Add one tablespoon of the olive oil to the skillet, add in the rolled meatballs, and cook the meatballs until cooked all the way through with no pink in the center. The middle needs to reach a Fahrenheit temperature of one-hundred and sixty-five degrees Fahrenheit. Be sure to stir the meatballs around occasionally so that all sides can cook!

- Once the meatballs are done cooking, remove and put them to the side for a while. Add the mushrooms and asparagus to the cooking pot, allowing them to cook until tender, about seven to nine minutes. Remove the skillet from the heat.

- In a medium-sized bowl, add the cooked pasta, meatballs, and vegetables along with the remaining Italian seasoning, one tablespoon of olive oil, and the balsamic vinegar. Toss all of the ingredients together and serve it warm, or chill it in the fridge before serving.

Greek Chicken Pita Sandwiches

For these pita sandwiches, be sure that you don't use whole-wheat or enriched pita bread, you want to use white pita bread as it is lowest in phosphorus and potassium. When making this recipe, please keep in mind that while this recipe uses onion and garlic powder, these are not the same as garlic and onion salt. These are different ingredients, as the powder contains much less sodium than the salt variety.

Chronic Kidney Disease Stage: 1-4

The Details:

The Number of Servings: 2

The Time Needed to Prepare: 5 minutes

The Time Required to Cook: 25 minutes

The Total Preparation/Cook Time: 30 minutes

Number of Calories In Individual Servings: 152

Protein Grams: 15

Phosphorus Milligrams: 257

Potassium Milligrams: 419

Sodium Milligrams: 65

Fat Grams: 5

Total Carbohydrates Grams: 9

Net Carbohydrates Grams: 7

The Ingredients:

- Chicken breast, cut into strips - .25 pound
- Onion powder - .25 teaspoon
- Black pepper, ground - .25 teaspoon
- Dill, dried - .5 teaspoon
- Parsley, dried – 1 teaspoon
- Garlic powder - .25 teaspoon
- Sesame seed oil - .5 teaspoon
- Cucumber, thinly sliced – 1
- Lettuce – 1 cup
- Pita bread – 2
- Hummus - .25 cup

The Instructions:

- Preheat your oven to a Fahrenheit temperature of four-hundred degrees.

- Place the chicken strips on a small baking sheet and toss them together with the onion powder, black pepper, dried dill, dried parsley, garlic powder, and sesame seed oil. Ensure that they are fully coated and then place it in the oven until the chicken strips are fully cooked. This should take twenty to twenty-five minutes. The middle of the chicken must reach a minimum Fahrenheit temperature of one-hundred and sixty-five degrees.

- Once the chicken is done cooking, remove it from the oven and prepare the remaining aspects of your sandwiches. You need to cut the pita breads in half and then open the pockets with your hands or a fork. Slice the cucumbers and tear the lettuce into bite-sized pieces.

- First, fill the pita bread halves with the lettuce, then the cucumber, and lastly, the cooked chicken strips. Serve it immediately to prevent the pita from going stale and while the chicken is still warm.

Chicken and Rice Soup

This soup is quick and easy to make and perfect for a cold winter day or for whenever you are feeling under the weather. However, keep in mind that you should plan this soup for on a day that you have other low-potassium meals planned. This is because while this soup is still classified as low-potassium, it does contain a little more potassium than many of the other recipes in this book.

While you can use low-sodium chicken broth from the store, you are best off using completely homemade broth so that you can ensure it has no added sodium.

Chronic Kidney Disease Stage: 1-4

The Details:

The Number of Servings: 2

The Time Needed to Prepare: 5 minutes

The Time Required to Cook: 25 minutes

The Total Preparation/Cook Time: 25 minutes

Number of Calories In Individual Servings: 374

Protein Grams: 19

Phosphorus Milligrams: 248

Potassium Milligrams: 649

Sodium Milligrams: 122

Fat Grams: 9

Total Carbohydrates Grams: 51

Net Carbohydrates Grams: 48

The Ingredients:

- Water – 2 cups
- Chicken broth, low-sodium – 1 cup
- Onion, dehydrated flakes – 1 tablespoon
- Garlic, minced – 4 cloves
- Celery, diced – 1 rib
- Carrots, sliced – 2
- Chicken breast, sliced into small cubes - .25 pound
- White rice, raw - .5 cup
- Poultry seasoning - .5 teaspoon
- Black pepper, ground - .25 teaspoon
- Olive oil – 1 tablespoon

The Instructions:

- Place the carrots, celery, garlic, and olive oil in a big casserole. Cook them over medium heat. Allow these to sauté together for five minutes and then add in the remaining ingredients. Stir the pot together well and bring it to a boil over medium-high heat.

- Once the pot comes to a boil, reduce it to a simmer, cover it with a lid, and allow it to cook until the rice and chicken are cooked about twenty minutes.

- Turn off the heat, allow the soup to sit for five minutes, and then serve.

Barbecue Tofu and Rice

This recipe makes faux-barbecue tofu. While barbecue sauce is not allowed on the kidney disease diet due to its high sodium and potassium contents, this recipe utilizes seasonings to make a similar barbecue flavor, but without the use of sodium or potassium-rich tomatoes. If you are a barbecue lover, you will absolutely love this tofu! Of course, you can also make it with chicken, if you wish.

This recipe makes use of onion powder and garlic powder; please keep in mind that these are very different from onion and garlic salt. Unlike the latter, these do not contain added sodium and can be used on the diet for kidney disease.

Chronic Kidney Disease Stage: 5/Dialysis

The Details:

The Number of Servings: 2

The Time Needed to Prepare: 5 minutes

The Time Required to Cook: 15 minutes

The Total Preparation/Cook Time: 20 minutes

Number of Calories In Individual Servings: 462

Protein Grams: 25

Phosphorus Milligrams: 368

Potassium Milligrams: 393

Sodium Milligrams: 23

Fat Grams: 20

Total Carbohydrates Grams: 46

Net Carbohydrates Grams: 44

The Ingredients:

- Tofu, extra firm, cut into bite-sized cubes – 16 ounces
- Corn starch – 1 tablespoon
- Red wine vinegar – 2 tablespoons
- Onion powder - .25 teaspoon
- Cayenne pepper - .125 teaspoon
- Smoked paprika - 1 teaspoon
- Brown sugar – 2 teaspoons
- Olive oil – 2 tablespoons
- Garlic powder - .25 teaspoon
- Black pepper, ground - .25 teaspoon
- Rice, white, cooked - .1.5 cups

The Instructions:

- Add the olive oil in a pan that is warmed over a heat of medium height. While you can use a stainless steel skillet, it is easier to use a non-stick skillet.

- In a medium-sized bowl, add in the corn starch, cayenne pepper, onion powder, smoked paprika, garlic powder, black ground pepper, and brown sugar. Whisk these together and then add in the tofu, tossing them together until the tofu is fully coated. Add in the red wine vinegar and toss the mixture together again.

- Place the tofu cubes in the hot oil of the skillet, giving them each a little space between the cubes so that they are not sticking. After a couple of minutes, flip them over and continue to do this until all sides of the cubes are golden in color. Remove the tofu from the skillet, and if you have any remaining uncooked cubes, cook them now as well.

- Serve the barbecue tofu over the white rice and enjoy!

Tex-Mex Quinoa Salad

This quinoa salad is simple to make, full of nutrients, and delicious! Enjoy it as a full meal either at home or on the road, as it travels well and can be enjoyed either warm or cold.

Chronic Kidney Disease Stage: 1-5/Dialysis

The Details:

The Number of Servings: 2

The Time Needed to Prepare: 5 minutes

The Time Required to Cook: 15 minutes

The Total Preparation/Cook Time: 20 minutes

Number of Calories In Individual Servings: 308

Protein Grams: 8

Phosphorus Milligrams: 252

Potassium Milligrams: 475

Sodium Milligrams: 31

Fat Grams: 12

Total Carbohydrates Grams: 43

Net Carbohydrates Grams: 38

The Ingredients:

- Water – 1 cup

- Olive oil – 1 teaspoon

- Garlic, minced – 2 cloves

- Quinoa, rinsed and drained - .5 cup
- Corn, canned, drained and rinsed - .5 cup
- Bell pepper, chopped - .5
- Green onion, sliced – 2
- Cilantro, fresh, chopped – 2 tablespoons
- Black beans, cooked – .5 cup
- Cumin - .25 teaspoon
- Lime juice – 1.5 tablespoons
- Black pepper, ground - .25 teaspoon
- Chili powder - .5 teaspoon
- Olive oil – 1 tablespoon
- Honey – 1 teaspoon

The Instructions:

6. In a saucepan over medium heat, cook the minced garlic in the single teaspoon of olive oil for one minute, until fragrant. Add in the water and quinoa and let the pot boiling. Simmer once boiling and cover the pot. Allow the quinoa to cook until all of the liquid has been absorbed, about fifteen minutes. Remove the quinoa from the heat.

7. While the quinoa cooks, prepare the vinaigrette by whisking together the remaining olive oil, honey, lime juice, cumin, chili powder, and black ground pepper.

8. Prepare a big-sized mixing dish where the cooked quinoa can be transferred and toss it together with the prepared vinaigrette, bell pepper, corn, and green onion until it is fully coated. Serve it warm or cold.

Chapter 6: Dinner

In this chapter, you will find recipes perfect for dinner whether you are eating a simple meal for one or a stunning meal for date night. You will love the recipes and how delicious they are.

Shepherd's Pie

This recipe is made with mashed cauliflower instead of potatoes, making it much lower in potassium than traditional Shepherd's pie. Not only that, but it is full of vegetables! In a single serving, you can get nearly half of your daily serving of vegetables.

Chronic Kidney Disease Stage: 1-4

The Details:

The Number of Servings: 2

The Time Needed to Prepare: 5 minutes

The Time Required to Cook: 35 minutes

The Total Preparation/Cook Time: 40 minutes

Number of Calories In Individual Servings: 210

Protein Grams: 14

Phosphorus Milligrams: 192

Potassium Milligrams: 632

Sodium Milligrams: 94

Fat Grams: 11

Total Carbohydrates Grams: 13

Net Carbohydrates Grams: 10

The Ingredients:

- Cauliflower, florets – 2 cups
- Turkey, ground - .25 pound
- Carrots, diced – 1
- Corn kernels - .25 cup
- Celery, diced – stalk
- Poultry seasoning – 1 teaspoon
- Black pepper, ground - .25 teaspoon
- Olive oil - .5 tablespoon

The Instructions:

- Place in a dish safe for microwave use with some water the cauliflower and cover it with a plate, and then microwave it until fork-tender. You can also steam it on the stove in a steam basket if you wish.

- While your cauliflower is steaming, allow the oven to preheat to a Fahrenheit temperature of four-hundred degrees.

- In a big-sized cooking pot, sauté the celery and carrots in the olive oil for five minutes. Add in the ground turkey and brown it until there is no pink remaining, about nine minutes. Stir in the corn, half of the black pepper, and three-quarters of the poultry seasoning.

- In a medium-sized kitchen bowl, mash the cauliflower with a hand-held potato masher until it is nice and creamy. Add in the remaining black pepper and poultry seasoning. Set aside the mashed cauliflower.

- Spread the meat and vegetable mixture into the bottom of a loaf pan. Spread the cauliflower evenly over the top, and then allow it to cook in the preheated oven for twenty minutes. If you want, you can turn the oven's broiler on the last two minutes to get the mashed cauliflower nice and golden.

Italian Herb Chicken and Asparagus

This dish is full of healthy protein from chicken and low in saturated fats. You will love the way that the herbed chicken pairs with the fresh asparagus and mild white rice. Enjoy it for either a high-protein lunch or dinner.

Chronic Kidney Disease Stage: 5/Dialysis

The Details:

The Number of Servings: 2

The Time Needed to Prepare: 5 minutes

The Time Required to Cook: 15 minutes

The Total Preparation/Cook Time: 20 minutes

Number of Calories In Individual Servings: 331

Protein Grams: 22

Phosphorus Milligrams: 259

Potassium Milligrams: 475

Sodium Milligrams: 38

Fat Grams: 9

Total Carbohydrates Grams: 38

Net Carbohydrates Grams: 36

The Ingredients:

- Chicken breast, cut into bite-sized pieces – .33 pound

- Italian herb seasoning – 2 teaspoon

- Black pepper, ground – .25 teaspoon

- Lemon zest - .25 teaspoon

- Garlic, minced – 3 cloves

- Olive oil – 1 tablespoon

- Asparagus, cut into bite-sized pieces - .33 pound

- Rice, white, cooked – 1.5 cups

The Instructions:

- Preheat your oven to a Fahrenheit temperature of four-hundred and fifty degrees before covering a large sheet pan with kitchen parchment.

- In a dish that is small in size, toss together the chicken, asparagus, herb seasoning, black pepper, lemon zest, garlic, and olive oil. You want to ensure that all of the ingredients are evenly coated. Either cook this mixture right away or allow it to marinate for fifteen minutes.

- Place the coated asparagus and chicken onto the baking pan and allow it to cook until the chicken reaches an internal Fahrenheit temperature of one-hundred and sixty-five degrees and the asparagus is tender about fifteen to twenty minutes.

- Remove the pan from the oven and either immediately serve it over the rice, or store it in the fridge or freezer to enjoy at a later date.

Baked Chicken Tacos

These chicken tacos are simple and easy to cook, as you just fill the tortillas with chicken mixture and then roast them. This gives you a slightly crispy taco shell that is much healthier than the fried alternative.

Chronic Kidney Disease Stage: 1-5/Dialysis

The Details:

The Number of Servings: 2

The Time Needed to Prepare: 5 minutes

The Time Required to Cook: 10 minutes

The Total Preparation/Cook Time: 15 minutes

Number of Calories In Individual Servings: 273

Protein Grams: 24

Phosphorus Milligrams: 423

Potassium Milligrams: 291

Sodium Milligrams: 76

Fat Grams: 9

Total Carbohydrates Grams: 22

Net Carbohydrates Grams: 19

The Ingredients:

- Corn tortillas – 4
- Chicken breast, cooked – 4 ounces
- Cheddar cheese, shredded, low-sodium - .33 cup
- Jalapeno, diced - .5

- Cumin - .25 teaspoon

- Chili powder - .25 teaspoon

- Lime juice – 2 teaspoons

The Instructions:

- Preheat your oven by setting it to a Fahrenheit temperature of four-hundred degrees. Meanwhile, microwave your tortillas for half a minute so that you can easily work with them without causing them to tear.

- Either dice the cooked chicken breast with a knife or shred it with a couple of forks. In a mixing dish, place together the cut chicken with the cheese, jalapeno, cumin, chili powder, and lime juice.

- Set your for tortillas on a baking sheet coated with kitchen parchment, and then fill them with the chicken and cheese mixture. Fold the tortillas in half, gently pressing them so that they stay folded. Place another baking sheet on top of the tacos, which will both keep them folded during the cooking process and act as an additional heat source to increase the crispiness of the tortilla.

- Bake the tacos in the preheated oven until they are golden-brown in color, about ten minutes. Watch them carefully, being careful not to allow them to burn.

- Remove the tacos from the oven immediately and serve them warm, either plain or with Greek yogurt in place of sour cream.

Mushroom Kale Quesadillas

These quesadillas are simple and easy to make and taste delicious! You will love the way that the mushrooms and kale perfectly complement the creamy cheese.

Chronic Kidney Disease Stage: 1-5/Dialysis

The Details:

The Number of Servings: 2

The Time Needed to Prepare: 5 minutes

The Time Required to Cook: 15 minutes

The Total Preparation/Cook Time: 20 minutes

Number of Calories In Individual Servings: 305

Protein Grams: 14

Phosphorus Milligrams: 462

Potassium Milligrams: 595

Sodium Milligrams: 24

Fat Grams: 15

Total Carbohydrates Grams: 30

Net Carbohydrates Grams: 26

The Ingredients:

- Tortillas, low-sodium, 8 inch – 4
- Olive oil – 1 tablespoon
- Mushrooms, sliced – 8 ounces

- Mozzarella cheese, shredded, low-sodium - .25 cup

- Cheddar cheese, shredded, low-sodium - .25 cup

- Kale, chopped – 3 cups

The Instructions:

11. Preheat your oven by setting it to a Fahrenheit temperature of four-hundred degrees and prepare a baking sheet by lining it with kitchen parchment.

12. Place the sliced mushrooms in a microwave-safe bowl and then soften them by cooking them in the microwave for three minutes. Drain off any liquid and then set them aside.

13. Using a pastry brush, coat both sides of all the tortillas with the olive oil, and then set two of them on the prepared baking sheet. Over both of the tortillas on the baking sheet divide the sliced mushrooms, kale, mozzarella cheese, and cheddar cheese. Place the remaining two tortillas on top of this mixture.

14. Place a baking sheet on top of the quesadillas and then place the two trays in the oven for twelve minutes, until the tortilla is golden and the cheese has melted. Remove the quesadillas from the oven, slice them up, and serve them alone or with a dollop of Greek yogurt.

Creamy Italian Chicken

This creamy dish is made healthy by using Greek yogurt in place of heavy cream, but it is still full of flavor thanks to the garlic and Parmesan cheese. Enjoy this chicken alongside your favorite grains and vegetables for a full meal.

Chronic Kidney Disease Stage: 1-5/Dialysis

The Details:

The Number of Servings: 2

The Time Needed to Prepare: 5 minutes

The Time Required to Cook: 15 minutes

The Total Preparation/Cook Time: 20 minutes

Number of Calories In Individual Servings: 225

Protein Grams: 20

Phosphorus Milligrams: 270

Potassium Milligrams: 419

Sodium Milligrams: 268

Fat Grams: 12

Total Carbohydrates Grams: 7

Net Carbohydrates Grams: 6

The Ingredients:

- Chicken breast, thinly sliced – 4 ounces
- Greek yogurt, plain - .25 cup
- Olive oil – 1 tablespoon

- Italian seasoning - .5 teaspoon

- Garlic powder - .5 teaspoon

- Parmesan cheese, grated - .25 cup

- Kale, chopped - .5 cup

- Bell pepper, thinly sliced – 1

- Water – 3 tablespoons

The Instructions:

- Into a large skillet, add the sliced chicken and olive oil over medium heat, cooking the slices until cooked through and golden brown, about seven to ten minutes. The internal temperature of the chicken must reach Fahrenheit one-hundred and sixty-five degrees.

- Remove the chicken from the pan and set it aside on a plate. Meanwhile, place the thinly sliced bell pepper, kale, Parmesan cheese, garlic powder, Italian seasoning, water, and the Greek yogurt into the pan. Cook this until the cheese is melted, it is warm, and just reaches a simmer.

- Place the chicken back into the simmering sauce and allow it to cook in the sauce for one minute before removing the dish from the heat.

Chicken and Rice Scampi

This chicken and rice scampi are creamy and full of flavor! It includes white wine, and the alcohol is cooked off during the cooking process. However, if you don't want to use white wine, you can use extra low-sodium chicken broth in its place.

Chronic Kidney Disease Stage: 1-5/Dialysis

The Details:

The Number of Servings: 2

The Time Needed to Prepare: 5 minutes

The Time Required to Cook: 15 minutes

The Total Preparation/Cook Time: 20 minutes

Number of Calories In Individual Servings: 403

Protein Grams: 20

Phosphorus Milligrams: 255

Potassium Milligrams: 324

Sodium Milligrams: 233

Fat Grams: 18

Total Carbohydrates Grams: 37

Net Carbohydrates Grams: 37

The Ingredients:

- Chicken breast, thinly sliced – 4 ounces
- Olive oil – 1 tablespoon
- Garlic powder - .25 teaspoon

- Black pepper, ground - .25 teaspoon

- Butter – 2 tablespoons

- Garlic, minced – 1 tablespoon

- Red pepper flakes - .25 teaspoon

- White wine, dry – 3 tablespoons

- White rice, cooked – 1.5 cup

- Parmesan cheese, grated – 3 tablespoons

- Greek yogurt, plain – 2 tablespoons

- Chicken broth, low-sodium – 3 tablespoons

The Instructions:

- Season your sliced chicken with the garlic powder and black ground pepper. Then, place it in a large skillet over medium heat along with the olive oil.

- Allow the chicken to sauté until it is cooked through and seared, about eight minutes. The internal temperature of the chicken must reach Fahrenheit one-hundred and sixty-five degrees. Remove the chicken from the skillet and set it aside on a plate.

- Add the butter, red pepper flakes, and minced garlic, and allow the garlic to cook for three minutes. Stir in the Greek yogurt, white wine, and chicken broth, stirring the mixture completely and allowing it to simmer for five minutes.

- Stir in the Parmesan cheese and place the chicken back in the pan, allowing it to simmer in the sauce for one minute.

- Remove the skillet from the heat and serve the chicken and sauce over the cooked white rice while still warm.

Mushroom Parmesan Pasta

With this creamy mushroom and Parmesan pasta dish, you won't miss traditional tomato sauces in the slightest! This sauce is much lower in potassium and phosphorus, but even more delicious. Enjoy this pasta alone, or with a side of homemade garlic bread.

Chronic Kidney Disease Stage: 1-5/Dialysis

The Details:

The Number of Servings: 2

The Time Needed to Prepare: 5 minutes

The Time Required to Cook: 15 minutes

The Total Preparation/Cook Time: 20 minutes

Number of Calories In Individual Servings: 398

Protein Grams: 14

Phosphorus Milligrams: 235

Potassium Milligrams: 374

Sodium Milligrams: 124

Fat Grams: 16

Total Carbohydrates Grams: 48

Net Carbohydrates Grams: 46

The Ingredients:

- Bowtie pasta – 4 ounces
- Olive oil – 2 tablespoons
- Mushrooms, sliced – 1 cup

- Garlic, minced – 1 tablespoon
- Onion, diced - .25 cup
- Chicken broth, low-sodium - .5 cup
- Greek yogurt, plain - .25 cup
- Parmesan cheese – 2 tablespoons
- Black pepper, ground - .25 teaspoon
- Kale, chopped – 1 cup

The Instructions:

1. Bring a pot of water to a boil and cook the pasta according to the directions on the package. Drain off the pasta water and set the pasta aside.

2. While the pasta cooks, in a large skillet, cook together the mushrooms, onions, and garlic in the olive oil until the mushrooms are soft and golden, about five to seven minutes. Add in the Greek yogurt, kale, black pepper, Parmesan cheese, and chicken broth. Cook the mixture for five more minutes until the kale is wilted and the sauce is simmering.

3. Toss together the pasta and the mushroom sauce, and then serve the dish immediately.

Stuffed Bell Pepper Soup

This soup is simple to make and delicious! You will love the stuffed bell pepper flavor, but made with much more ease. This soup is easy to cook and only tastes better once it has a chance to chill in the fridge overnight allowing the flavors to meld. That means you can enjoy one serving for dinner and enjoy another serving from lunch the following day.

Chronic Kidney Disease Stage: 1-5/Dialysis

The Details:

The Number of Servings: 2

The Time Needed to Prepare: 5 minutes

The Time Required to Cook: 20 minutes

The Total Preparation/Cook Time: 25 minutes

Number of Calories In Individual Servings: 283

Protein Grams: 16

Phosphorus Milligrams: 183

Potassium Milligrams: 369

Sodium Milligrams: 85

Fat Grams: 9

Total Carbohydrates Grams: 32

Net Carbohydrates Grams: 30

The Ingredients:

- Chicken broth, low-sodium – 2 cups
- Bell pepper, red, diced – 1

- Garlic, minced – 4 cloves

- Onion, diced - .5 cup

- Ground turkey – 4 ounces

- Olive oil – 2 teaspoons

- Italian seasoning – 1 teaspoon

- White rice, cooked – 1 cup

- Parsley, fresh, chopped – 1 tablespoon

The Instructions:

1. In a large pan over medium heat, cook the ground turkey with the olive oil, onion, and garlic until the turkey is fully cooked and no pink is remaining about five to seven minutes.

2. Add the black pepper, Italian seasoning, and bell pepper to the soup pot, allowing it to cook for three more minutes.

3. Into the pot, pour the low-sodium chicken broth, simmer the soup for fifteen minutes, until the bell peppers are tender. Stir in the cooked rice and parsley before serving.

Seared Chicken and Green Beans

This chicken is delicious and simple to make, and it perfectly pairs with the fresh lemon green beans. Enjoy this chicken alongside your favorite grains for a complete meal.

Chronic Kidney Disease Stage: 1-5/Dialysis

The Details:

The Number of Servings: 2

The Time Needed to Prepare: 5 minutes

The Time Required to Cook: 15 minutes

The Total Preparation/Cook Time: 20 minutes

Number of Calories In Individual Servings: 160

Protein Grams: 14

Phosphorus Milligrams: 156

Potassium Milligrams: 385

Sodium Milligrams: 37

Fat Grams: 8

Total Carbohydrates Grams: 7

Net Carbohydrates Grams: 5

The Ingredients:

- Chicken breast – 4 ounces
- Green beans, trimmed – .25 pound
- Garlic, minced – 3 cloves

- Olive oil – 1 tablespoon
- Paprika - .25 teaspoon
- Onion powder - .25 teaspoon
- Black pepper, ground - .25 teaspoon
- Lemon juice – 1 tablespoon
- Chicken broth, low-sodium – 2 tablespoons
- Water - .25 cup
- Red chili flakes - .25 teaspoon
- Parsley, fresh, chopped – 3 tablespoons

The Instructions:

1. Season the chicken with the onion powder, black pepper, and paprika, and then set it aside.

2. Meanwhile, place the green beans in a microwave-safe bowl along with the water. Steam the green beans in the microwave for eight minutes until they are almost cooked but still a little crisp.

3. In a large skillet, cook the seasoned chicken in the olive oil until it is cooked all the way through, about seven to ten minutes. The chicken is only done cooking once it reaches an internal Fahrenheit temperature of one-hundred and sixty-five degrees. Remove the chicken from the skillet and set it aside.

4. Into the skillet add the garlic, parsley, chili flakes, and the microwaved green beans. Allow them to cook for an additional four minutes until

they are tender to your preference. Add in the lemon juice, chicken broth, and cooked chicken, allowing the sauce to simmer for two to three minutes.

5. Remove the skillet from the heat and serve immediately with a side of grains or bread.

Poached Thai Salmon

This poached salmon is full of Thai flavors such as lemongrass, ginger, and garlic. You will love the flavor, especially when it is served with freshly cooked rice. Try topping the rice with a little extra lime juice for added flavor.

Chronic Kidney Disease Stage: 1-5/Dialysis

The Details:

The Number of Servings: 2

The Time Needed to Prepare: 5 minutes

The Time Required to Cook: 15 minutes

The Total Preparation/Cook Time: 20 minutes

Number of Calories In Individual Servings: 250

Protein Grams: 18

Phosphorus Milligrams: 257

Potassium Milligrams: 446

Sodium Milligrams: 108

Fat Grams: 16

Total Carbohydrates Grams: 8

Net Carbohydrates Grams: 7

The Ingredients:

- Salmon fillets – 6 ounces
- Black pepper, ground - .25 teaspoon
- Olive oil – 1 tablespoon

- Garlic, minced – 2 cloves

- Ginger powder – 1 teaspoon

- Lemongrass, peeled and grated – 1 tablespoon

- Brown sugar – 2 teaspoons

- Red chili flakes – 1 teaspoon

- Coconut milk – 3 tablespoons

- Lime juice – 2 teaspoons

- Lime zest - .25 teaspoon

The Instructions:

1. Season the salmon with the black pepper and then sear it in a skillet over medium-high heat in the olive oil. Cook the salmon skin-side up at first, then after one to two minutes, flip it over and cook the skin-side down for one minute. Remove the salmon from the skillet and place it on a plate.

2. Reduce the heat of the skillet to medium-low and add in the lemongrass and garlic, allowing them to cook until golden, about one minute. Add in the sugar, ground ginger, and red pepper flakes, about thirty seconds until caramelized.

3. Stir in the coconut milk, deglazing the pan in the process. Add the salmon back into the sauce and allow it to gently simmer until cooked, about four minutes.

4. Add the lime juice and zest to the skillet, and serve it with either rice or noodles.

The Best Turkey Burgers

These burgers are not only delicious, but they are also incredibly simple! You can serve them alongside a bed of rice, wrapped in lettuce, with store-bought low-sodium buns, or you can even make your own buns. Try turning the Fluffy Sandwich Bread or the French Bread from later on in this book into hamburger buns and you will not be disappointed!

Chronic Kidney Disease Stage: 1-5/Dialysis

The Details:

The Number of Servings: 2

The Time Needed to Prepare: 5 minutes

The Time Required to Cook: 15 minutes

The Total Preparation/Cook Time: 20 minutes

Number of Calories In Individual Servings: 130

Protein Grams: 11

Phosphorus Milligrams: 129

Potassium Milligrams: 206

Sodium Milligrams: 37

Fat Grams: 8

Total Carbohydrates Grams: 3

Net Carbohydrates Grams: 3

The Ingredients:

- Turkey, ground - .25 pound
- Garlic, minced – 2 cloves

- Onion, diced - .25 cup

- Parsley, fresh, chopped – 2 tablespoons

- Mustard seed, ground - .25 teaspoon

- Red pepper flakes - .25 teaspoon

- Black pepper, ground - .125 teaspoon

- Olive oil - .5 tablespoon

The Instructions:

1. In a bowl, lightly knead together the ground turkey, onion, garlic, parsley, and spices. Be careful to not over mix the meat, otherwise, it becomes tough. You only want to mix it just until combined.

2. Use your hands to form the meat into two patties of even thickness. You want to make them slightly larger than the buns since the meat will shrink as it cooks.

3. Grease a skillet with the olive oil and pan fry the patties over medium heat until they are cooked through with an internal temperature of one-hundred and sixty-five degrees Fahrenheit. You can also cook them under your oven's broiler or on the grill for the best flavor.

Chapter 7: Side Dishes

These side dishes can complement any meal. Whether you have made an elaborate entree or are eating a simple slice of chicken, you can enjoy these side dishes to both increase the flavor and the nutrition. You will find both grain and vegetable-based side dishes in this chapter, ensuring that you have something for every occasion.

Lime Cilantro Rice

Rice is a wonderful way to bulk up your meals and add needed calories, without adding too much excess phosphorus, potassium, or sodium. This rice is particularly tasty, as it is full of lime and cilantro, making it a wonderful option whenever you want to enjoy a fresh dish or Tex-Mex.

Chronic Kidney Disease Stage: 1-5/Dialysis

The Details:

The Number of Servings: 2

The Time Needed to Prepare: 5 minutes

The Time Required to Cook: 20 minutes

The Total Preparation/Cook Time: 25 minutes

Number of Calories In Individual Servings: 363

Protein Grams: 5

Phosphorus Milligrams: 74

Potassium Milligrams: 86

Sodium Milligrams: 5

Fat Grams: 10

Total Carbohydrates Grams: 60

Net Carbohydrates Grams: 58

The Ingredients:

- White rice – .75 cup
- Water – 1.5 cups
- Olive oil – 1.5 tablespoons
- Bay leaf, ground - .25 teaspoon
- Lime juice – 1 tablespoon
- Lemon juice – 1 tablespoon
- Lime zest - .25 teaspoon
- Cilantro, chopped - .25 cup

The Instructions:

1. Place the white rice and water in a medium-sized saucepan and bring it to a boil over medium heat. Reduce the heat to a light simmer and cover the pot with a lid, allowing it to cook until all of the water has been absorbed about eighteen to twenty minutes.

2. Once the rice is done cooking, stir in the ground bay leaf, olive oil, lime juice, lemon juice, lime zest, and cilantro. You want to do this with a fork, preferably, as this will fluff the rice rather than causing it to compact. Serve while warm.

Spanish Rice

Unlike most Spanish rice, this one does not contain tomatoes. However, it is still high on flavors and you will find it is the perfect addition for tacos, burritos, and simply as a side dish whenever you crave a burst of flavor.

Chronic Kidney Disease Stage: 1-5/Dialysis

The Details:

The Number of Servings: 2

The Time Needed to Prepare: 5 minutes

The Time Required to Cook: 20 minutes

The Total Preparation/Cook Time: 25 minutes

Number of Calories In Individual Servings: 303

Protein Grams: 6

Phosphorus Milligrams: 104

Potassium Milligrams: 197

Sodium Milligrams: 57

Fat Grams: 1

Total Carbohydrates Grams: 65

Net Carbohydrates Grams: 63

The Ingredients:

- White rice – .75 cup

- Chicken broth, low sodium– 1.5 cups

- Onion dehydrated flakes – 2 tablespoons

- Garlic, minced – 2 cloves

- Lemon juice – 1 tablespoon

- Cumin, ground - .25 teaspoon

- Chili powder - .5 teaspoon

- Oregano, dried - .5 teaspoon

- Black pepper, ground - .25 teaspoon

- Cilantro, chopped – 3 tablespoons

The Instructions:

1. Place the rice, chicken broth, onion flakes, and minced garlic in a medium-sized saucepan. Bring the chicken broth and rice to a boil over medium heat, and then reduce the heat to a light simmer, cover it with a lid, and allow it to cook until the liquid has all been absorbed about eighteen to twenty minutes.

2. Use a fork to fluff the rice mix in the lemon juice, cumin, chili powder, oregano, black pepper, and cilantro. Once combined, serve the rice while still warm.

Parmesan Quinoa with Peas

This Parmesan quinoa might be higher in minerals than rice dishes, however, if you have a little extra room for phosphorus and potassium in your daily allotment, you will love the addition of this dish! This dish is great when you need a little extra protein, or simply want an easy side dish that feels fancy.

Chronic Kidney Disease Stage: 1-5/Dialysis

The Details:

The Number of Servings: 2

The Time Needed to Prepare: 5 minutes

The Time Required to Cook: 20 minutes

The Total Preparation/Cook Time: 25 minutes

Number of Calories In Individual Servings: 386

Protein Grams: 13

Phosphorus Milligrams: 378

Potassium Milligrams: 465

Sodium Milligrams: 144

Fat Grams: 16

Total Carbohydrates Grams: 47

Net Carbohydrates Grams: 41

The Ingredients:

- Quinoa – .75 cup

- Water – 1.5 cups

- Green peas, thawed if frozen - .75 cup

- Black pepper, ground - .25 teaspoon

- Olive oil – 1.5 tablespoons

- Parmesan cheese, grated – 3 tablespoons

The Instructions:

1. Place the uncooked quinoa in a fine metal sieve and rinse it well with water until there is no debris running off.

2. Place the quinoa and water in a medium-sized metal saucepan and bring it to a boil over medium heat. Once it attains a boil, reduce it to a light simmer, cover the pot with a lid, and allow it to cook until the water has all been absorbed. This should take fifteen to twenty minutes.

3. Remove the quinoa from the heat and allow it to sit with the lid on for five minutes. Once it has set, use a fork to fluff the quinoa and stir in the green peas, olive oil, and quinoa. Close the lid once again, allowing it to sit for five additional minutes to warm the peas and melt the cheese. Enjoy the quinoa while warm.

Mushroom Orzo

Orzo is a type of pasta formed in the shape of rice. It has a wonderful flavor and texture, and due to the small sizes, it greatly absorbs the flavor of whatever it is cooked. You will love this orzo with the addition of mushrooms, garlic, and sage.

Chronic Kidney Disease Stage: 1-5/Dialysis

The Details:

The Number of Servings: 2

The Time Needed to Prepare: 5 minutes

The Time Required to Cook: 20 minutes

The Total Preparation/Cook Time: 25 minutes

Number of Calories In Individual Servings: 337

Protein Grams: 18

Phosphorus Milligrams: 63

Potassium Milligrams: 430

Sodium Milligrams: 43

Fat Grams: 8

Total Carbohydrates Grams: 99

Net Carbohydrates Grams: 95

The Ingredients:

- Orzo - .75 cup
- Chicken broth, low-sodium – 1.25 cup
- Mushrooms, diced – 4 ounces

- Garlic, minced – 3 cloves

- Onion flakes, dehydrated – 1 tablespoon

- Olive oil – 1 tablespoon

- Sage, ground - .25 teaspoon

The Instructions:

1. Place the diced mushrooms, olive oil, and garlic in a medium-sized metal saucepan and allow them to sauté over medium heat for five minutes. Add in the sage, onion flakes, orzo, and low-sodium chicken broth. Bring the mixture to a boil.

2. Reduce the heat of the skillet to a light simmer, cover the pot with a lid, and allow it to cook until all of the liquid has been absorbed about nine minutes. Fluff the orzo with a fork before serving.

Carrot and Pineapple Slaw

This slaw is sweet and savory with the pineapple and grapes perfectly complementing the carrots. You will especially love that this slaw can be made up to a day in advance, making it the perfect side dish to take with you to work, on a road trip, or to a potluck.

Chronic Kidney Disease Stage: 1-5/Dialysis

The Details:

The Number of Servings: 2

The Time Needed to Prepare: 5 minutes

The Time Required to Cook: 0 minutes

The Total Preparation/Cook Time: 5 minutes

Number of Calories In Individual Servings: 264

Protein Grams: 2

Phosphorus Milligrams: 74

Potassium Milligrams: 423

Sodium Milligrams: 91

Fat Grams: 17

Total Carbohydrates Grams: 29

Net Carbohydrates Grams: 25

The Ingredients:

- Carrot matchsticks – 5 ounces
- Pineapple chunks, canned, liquid drained - .5 cup
- Grapes, sliced in half - .5 cup

- Pecan pieces - .25 cup

- Mayonnaise, low-sodium - .33 cup

- Lemon juice – 1 tablespoon

The Instructions:

1. In a bowl, toss together the carrot matchsticks, drained pineapple chunks, sliced grapes, and pecan pieces. Stir in the low-sodium mayonnaise and lemon juice.

2. Cover the bowl with plastic wrap or a lid and then allow it to chill and marinate for at least an hour before serving. You can make this slaw up to a day in advance.

Sesame Cucumber Salad

This is a take on a popular dish throughout East Asia, although this version does not use soy sauce which is high in sodium and other minerals. However, this salad is still full of flavor, making it the perfect refreshing dish to enjoy in the summer months.

Chronic Kidney Disease Stage: 1-5/Dialysis

The Details:

The Number of Servings: 2

The Time Needed to Prepare: 5 minutes

The Time Required to Cook: 0 minutes

The Total Preparation/Cook Time: 5 minutes

Number of Calories In Individual Servings: 92

Protein Grams: 1

Phosphorus Milligrams: 46

Potassium Milligrams: 250

Sodium Milligrams: 117

Fat Grams: 5

Total Carbohydrates Grams: 9

Net Carbohydrates Grams: 8

The Ingredients:

- Cucumbers, thinly sliced – 1
- Sesame seeds - .5 teaspoon
- Rice wine vinegar – 1 tablespoon

- Sugar - .5 tablespoon

- Sesame seed oil – 1.5 tablespoons

- Red pepper flakes - .25 teaspoon

The Instructions:

1. You want the cucumbers sliced as thinly as you can get them. While you can certainly do this with a knife, it is quicker and easier if you use a mandolin.

2. In a medium to a small bowl, whisk together the sesame seeds, rice wine vinegar, sugar, sesame seed oil, and red pepper flakes. Once well combined, add in the cucumbers and toss the vegetables in the vinaigrette. Serve immediately.

Creamy Jalapeno Corn

This creamy jalapeno corn is the perfect treat for the summer, especially when paired with grilled foods. Try this corn alongside grilled chicken or turkey burgers, and you will absolutely love it!

Chronic Kidney Disease Stage: 1-5/Dialysis

The Details:

The Number of Servings: 2

The Time Needed to Prepare: 5 minutes

The Time Required to Cook: 15 minutes

The Total Preparation/Cook Time: 20 minutes

Number of Calories In Individual Servings: 284

Protein Grams: 7

Phosphorus Milligrams: 200

Potassium Milligrams: 293

Sodium Milligrams: 82

Fat Grams: 19

Total Carbohydrates Grams: 20

Net Carbohydrates Grams: 18

The Ingredients:

- Corn kernels, fresh – 1 cup
- Red bell pepper, diced - .25 cup
- Jalapeno, seeded and diced – 1

- Cream cheese – 1.5 ounces

- Olive oil – 1 tablespoon

- Black pepper, ground - .25 teaspoon

- Cheddar cheese, low-sodium - .25 cup

The Instructions:

1. Preheat your oven to a Fahrenheit temperature of three-hundred and fifty degrees.

2. In a medium saucepan, sauté the bell pepper and jalapeno in the olive oil until softened, about four minutes. Add in the cream cheese and continue to stir until it melts and combines with the vegetables.

3. Add in the corn, black pepper, and half of the cheese. After the mixture is combined, sprinkle the remaining cheese over the top and place the saucepan in the oven to cook until it is hot and bubbling about fifteen minutes.

Crispy Parmesan Cauliflower

This cauliflower is coated in Parmesan cheese and breadcrumbs for a flavorful and crispy coating, allowing you to enjoy a savory treat. If you are someone who has a weakness for French fries, you will also love this cauliflower.

Chronic Kidney Disease Stage: 1-5/Dialysis

The Details:

The Number of Servings: 2

The Time Needed to Prepare: 5 minutes

The Time Required to Cook: 30 minutes

The Total Preparation/Cook Time: 35 minutes

Number of Calories In Individual Servings: 106

Protein Grams: 5

Phosphorus Milligrams: 166

Potassium Milligrams: 369

Sodium Milligrams: 222

Fat Grams: 9

Total Carbohydrates Grams: 16

Net Carbohydrates Grams: 14

The Ingredients:

- Cauliflower florets – 2 cups
- Black pepper, ground - .125 teaspoon
- Garlic, minced – 2 cloves

- Parmesan cheese, grated – 2 tablespoons

- Bread crumbs, plain - .25 cup

- Olive oil – 1 tablespoon

The Instructions:

1. Preheat your oven to a Fahrenheit temperature of four-hundred degrees and line a baking sheet with kitchen parchment.

2. In one small bowl, combine the olive oil and the garlic. In another, combine the Parmesan cheese, bread crumbs, and black pepper.

3. Dip the cauliflower piece-by-piece first into the olive oil mixture, and then into the bread crumb mixture. After you coat each piece, set it on the kitchen parchment-lined sheet.

4. Place the cauliflower sheet in the middle of the oven and roast the cauliflower until it reaches golden brown perfection, about thirty minutes. Serve it immediately, while it is still warm and crispy.

Cucumber Dill Salad with Greek Yogurt Dressing

This creamy dill salad is full of refreshing flavors, making it ideal to enjoy alongside savory meals. Whether you are eating a light meal of fish or a heavier meal, you will find that this salad with the fresh dill and zesty Greek yogurt complements anything savory.

Chronic Kidney Disease Stage: 1-5/Dialysis

The Details:

The Number of Servings: 2

The Time Needed to Prepare: 5 minutes

The Time Required to Cook: 0 minutes

The Total Preparation/Cook Time: 5 minutes

Number of Calories In Individual Servings: 106

Protein Grams: 5

Phosphorus Milligrams: 166

Potassium Milligrams: 369

Sodium Milligrams: 222

Fat Grams: 9

Total Carbohydrates Grams: 16

Net Carbohydrates Grams: 14

The Ingredients:

- Cucumbers, cut thinly – 2
- Red onion, small, thinly sliced - .5

- Greek yogurt, plain – 3 tablespoons

- Honey – 2 teaspoons

- White vinegar – 4 teaspoons

- Black pepper, ground - .125 teaspoon

- Garlic powder - .125 teaspoon

- Dill, fresh, chopped – 1.5 tablespoons

The Instructions:

1. Use either a knife or a mandolin to cut the cucumbers into thin and even slices, about .25 of an inch thick.

2. In a medium bowl, whisk together the fresh dill, garlic powder, black pepper, white vinegar, honey, and Greek yogurt.

3. Into the bowl with the prepared Greek yogurt dressing, add the cucumbers and red onion, and toss them together until fully coated. Cover the bowl with a lid or plastic wrap and allow it to chill in the fridge for at least an hour before enjoying. You can make this salad up to a day in advance.

Zesty Green Beans with Almonds

These green beans are full of flavor from zesty lemon, shallot, and garlic, which is perfectly complemented by the nutty and creamy sliced almonds. These green beans may be simple, but they feel extraordinary.

Chronic Kidney Disease Stage: 1-5/Dialysis

The Details:

The Number of Servings: 2

The Time Needed to Prepare: 5 minutes

The Time Required to Cook: 10 minutes

The Total Preparation/Cook Time: 15 minutes

Number of Calories In Individual Servings: 143

Protein Grams: 3

Phosphorus Milligrams: 84

Potassium Milligrams: 322

Sodium Milligrams: 8

Fat Grams: 10

Total Carbohydrates Grams: 11

Net Carbohydrates Grams: 8

The Ingredients:

- Green beans, trimmed - .5 pound

- Olive oil – 1 tablespoon

- Shallot, diced – 1

- Garlic, minced – 2 cloves

- Almonds, sliced – 2 tablespoons

- Lemon zest - .25 teaspoon

- Lemon juice – 1 teaspoon

- Black pepper, ground - .125 teaspoon

The Instructions:

1. In a large skillet, sauté the shallot and garlic in the olive oil over medium heat until soft, about three minutes. Add in the green beans and black pepper and continue to cook the green beans until they are tender about seven minutes.

2. Once the green beans are ready, stir in the lemon juice and lemon zest, and then top the skillet off with the sliced almonds.

Roasted Carrots and Broccoli

These vegetables are roasted to perfection, allowing you to enjoy the sweet and savory pair of carrots and broccoli. These vegetables are not only full of flavor but also nutrients, making them a wonderful choice to add to your meal plan.

Chronic Kidney Disease Stage: 1-5/Dialysis

The Details:

The Number of Servings: 2

The Time Needed to Prepare: 5 minutes

The Time Required to Cook: 20 minutes

The Total Preparation/Cook Time: 25 minutes

Number of Calories In Individual Servings: 184

Protein Grams: 4

Phosphorus Milligrams: 100

Potassium Milligrams: 494

Sodium Milligrams: 86

Fat Grams: 14

Total Carbohydrates Grams: 12

Net Carbohydrates Grams: 8

The Ingredients:

- Broccoli Florets - .5 pound
- Carrot, large, cut on the bias – 1
- Olive oil – 2 tablespoons

- Garlic, minced – 2 cloves

- Lemon zest - .5 tablespoon

- Parmesan cheese – .5 tablespoon

- Lemon juice - .5 tablespoon

- Black pepper, ground - .125 teaspoon

The Instructions:

- Preheat your oven to a Fahrenheit temperature of four-hundred and fifty degrees.

- In a bowl, toss together the black pepper, garlic, olive oil, chopped carrot, and broccoli florets. Spread the vegetable mixture onto a baking sheet.

- Roast the vegetables until they are tender and lightly browned, about fifteen to twenty minutes. Remove the pan from the stove, transfer them back to the bowl from earlier, and toss them with the lemon zest, lemon juice, and grated Parmesan cheese. Enjoy the vegetables while still warm.

Tahini and Pomegranate Carrots

These carrots are extravagant enough to enjoy on Thanksgiving or Christmas, but easy enough to cook any day of the week. Enjoy these carrots whether you wish to wow a crowd or enjoy a rich and flavorful treat.

Chronic Kidney Disease Stage: 1-5/Dialysis

The Details:

The Number of Servings: 2

The Time Needed to Prepare: 5 minutes

The Time Required to Cook: 30 minutes

The Total Preparation/Cook Time: 35 minutes

Number of Calories In Individual Servings: 143

Protein Grams: 2

Phosphorus Milligrams: 102

Potassium Milligrams: 434

Sodium Milligrams: 88

Fat Grams: 9

Total Carbohydrates Grams: 14

Net Carbohydrates Grams: 10

The Ingredients:

- Carrots - .5 pound
- Olive oil – 2 teaspoons
- Tahini paste – 1 tablespoon

- Cilantro, chopped – 1 tablespoon

- Cumin seeds - .5 teaspoon

- Black pepper, ground - .125 teaspoon

- Pomegranate arils – 2 tablespoons

The Instructions:

- Set the oven to a Fahrenheit temperature of three-hundred and seventy-five.

- In a bowl, toss together the whole carrots with the olive oil, cumin seeds, and black pepper. Place them on a baking sheet and allow them to roast until tender, about thirty minutes.

- Remove the carrots from the oven and drizzle the tahini over them, and then sprinkle both the cilantro and the pomegranate arils over the top before serving.

Chapter 8: Breads

In this chapter, you will find all the breads your heart might wish for. Unlike the breads commonly sold on the market, these are all low-sodium, allowing you to enjoy them to your heart's content. Whether you are craving something savory or sweet, you are sure to find what you wish for here.

Fluffy Sandwich Bread

This bread is perfect for sandwiches, as it is light, fluffy, and rich. Not only is it good for sandwiches, but you can also enjoy it for breakfast as toast.

Chronic Kidney Disease Stage: 1-5/Dialysis

The Details:

The Number of Servings: 5

The Time Needed to Prepare: 15 minutes

The Time Required to Cook: 30 minutes

The Total Preparation/Cook Time: 45 minutes

Number of Calories In Individual Servings: 371

Protein Grams: 8

Phosphorus Milligrams: 95

Potassium Milligrams: 122

Sodium Milligrams: 45

Fat Grams: 8

Total Carbohydrates Grams: 64

Net Carbohydrates Grams: 62

The Ingredients:

- Almond milk, warm – 1 cup
- Olive oil – 2 tablespoons
- Honey – 1 tablespoon
- Active dry yeast – 1 packet
- All-purpose flour – 3 cups
- Butter, melted – 1 tablespoon

The Instructions:

1. Place the milk, honey, and yeast into the bowl of your stand mixer, whisking them together until the yeast is completely dissolved. Allow this to sit in a warm place for five to ten minutes, until the yeast is especially foamy and bubbly.

2. Once the yeast is bubbly, add in the all-purpose flour and olive oil. Add the hook attachment onto your stand mixer and knead the dough until it is smooth and pulls away from the sides of the bowl, about ten minutes. Be sure that the stand mixer is on low speed.

3. Cover the bowl of the stand mixer with a clean kitchen towel, and allow it to rise in a warm place until it doubles in size, about an hour.

4. Once the dough has risen, punch it down and place it in a loaf pan, greased with olive oil.

Cover this pan back up with the clean towel and allow it to rise once more in a warm location until doubled in size, about forty-five minutes.

5. Bake your risen bread loaf in an oven preheated to three-hundred and twenty-five degrees until it is cooked through, about twenty-five to thirty minutes. Once the loaf is removed from the oven, use a pastry brush and coat the top of the loaf with melted butter.

No-Knead Rustic Loaf

This loaf is incredibly simple, yet resembles the rustic gourmet loaves from Italy and France. Enjoy this loaf as a simple sandwich, grilled panini, morning toast, or even to make bread crumbs to cook with.

Chronic Kidney Disease Stage: 1-5/Dialysis

The Details:

The Number of Servings: 4

The Time Needed to Prepare: 10 minutes

The Time Required to Cook: 45 minutes

The Total Preparation/Cook Time: 55 minutes

Number of Calories In Individual Servings: 346

Protein Grams: 10

Phosphorus Milligrams: 111

Potassium Milligrams: 115

Sodium Milligrams: 4

Fat Grams: 1

Total Carbohydrates Grams: 72

Net Carbohydrates Grams: 70

The Ingredients:

- All-purpose flour – 3 cups
- Active dry yeast – 1.5 teaspoons
- Water, warm – 1.5 cups

The Instructions:

1. In a large bowl, combine the flour and yeast, and then add the flour and combine it with a spoon until it forms a thick dough. This dough will likely stick to the bottom of the bowl which is okay.

2. Cover your bowl with a clean kitchen towel, and allow it to rise in a warm location until doubled about two to three hours.

3. Set your oven to a Fahrenheit temperature of four-hundred and fifty degrees. While you can use a standard aluminum pan; if you have a pizza stone, you can set this in the oven to warm for forty-five minutes before using. Fill a small dish with two inches of water and place it at the bottom of your oven. Don't skip this step, as the steam from the water creates a crispy crust.

4. Sprinkle some flour onto a clean cutting board and place your bread loaf on it. Use your hands to form the bread into a round ball, without kneading. Use a sharp knife and score the top of the load with a large knife.

5. Place the dough onto the hot pizza stone or a prepared aluminum pan and place it in the oven to cook until golden brown, crisp, and cooked through, about forty-five minutes. Once done cooking, allow the loaf to cool completely before cutting.

Pita Bread

Whereas pita bread you buy in the store can contain a decent amount of sodium, this homemade pita bread only contains three milligrams! That means you can enjoy pita as much as you would like, allowing you to make simple sandwiches or more complex Indian meals.

Chronic Kidney Disease Stage: 1-5/Dialysis

The Details:

The Number of Servings: 4

The Time Needed to Prepare: 30 minutes

The Time Required to Cook: 30 minutes

The Total Preparation/Cook Time: 60 minutes

Number of Calories In Individual Servings: 272

Protein Grams: 8

Phosphorus Milligrams: 91

Potassium Milligrams: 97

Sodium Milligrams: 3

Fat Grams: 0

Total Carbohydrates Grams: 56

Net Carbohydrates Grams: 54

The Ingredients:

- All-purpose flour – 3.5 cups
- Water, warm – 1.25 cups
- Active dry yeast – 1 tablespoon

The Instructions:

1. In your stand mixer bowl, combine the warm water, yeast, and half of the all-purpose flour to form a soft batter. Continue to add the remaining all-purpose flour until you get a soft dough that doesn't stick to the sides of the bowl. Continue to knead the dough with the hook attachment on low speed for four to five minutes. If you are kneading by hand, you will need to knead it for double the time.

2. Place the dough on a clean floured surface and separate it into six portions of equal size. Roll each portion into the shape of a ball. Cover all six of the dough balls with a clean kitchen towel and allow them to rise for fifteen minutes.

3. Using a rolling pin, roll each ball into a disk about .25 inch thick. Try to keep each disk of dough the same thickness all the way through so that it cooks evenly. Allow the rolled out dough disks rise for thirty to forty minutes while covered with a clean kitchen towel. You know that they are ready when they are slightly puffy.

4. While the pita disks rise allow your oven to preheat to a Fahrenheit temperature of four-hundred and twenty-five degrees. Prepare a baking sheet by coating it with kitchen parchment.

5. Once the oven is done preheating and the pita disks have risen, transfer two of them onto the prepared baking sheet. Flip the pita disks over,

so that the bottom side of the disk that had been resting on the counter is now facing upward. Spritz the dough disks with clean water.

6. Allow the pita disks to bake in the oven until they are lightly browned and have puffed up by several inches, about ten minutes. Sometimes, pita will refuse to puff up, and that's okay, too, you can use these as a flatbread.

7. Continue to bake the remaining pita dough after the first two are removed from the oven.

Italian Focaccia

This simple Italian Focaccia doesn't require kneading or the use of a stand mixer. You can easily make it with little hands-on work, allowing you to make a delicious and luxurious meal even if you have little time or energy to spare.

Chronic Kidney Disease Stage: 1-5/Dialysis

The Details:

The Number of Servings: 4

The Time Needed to Prepare: 15 minutes

The Time Required to Cook: 25 minutes

The Total Preparation/Cook Time: 40 minutes

Number of Calories In Individual Servings: 295

Protein Grams: 7

Phosphorus Milligrams: 74

Potassium Milligrams: 118

Sodium Milligrams: 59

Fat Grams: 7

Total Carbohydrates Grams: 49

Net Carbohydrates Grams: 48

The Ingredients:

- All-purpose flour – 2 cups

- Yeast – 1.25 teaspoons

- Warm water – 1 cup

- Olive oil – 2 tablespoons

- Italian herb seasoning – 1 teaspoon

- Garlic, minced – 3 cloves

The Instructions:

1. In a large bowl, combine the all-purpose flour and yeast, stirring well to incorporate the yeast evenly. Add in the warm water and continue to stir the mixture until the water and flour are completely combined. Cover the bowl with plastic wrap and allow the dough to chill in the refrigerator for at least eight hours, but up to twenty-four hours.

2. Grease a nine-inch round baking pan and then line it with kitchen parchment. Pour one tablespoon of your olive oil into the center of the lined pan. Add the dough into the pan, turning it over and coating it with the oil from the pan. Form a dough ball and then wrap the pan with plastic wrap, allowing it to rise in a warm location for two hours.

3. Preheat your oven to a Fahrenheit temperature of four-hundred and fifty degrees.

4. Drizzle the remaining tablespoon of olive oil over the dough ball, and then use your fingers to press the dough straight down into the pan. As you do this, you should create dimples in the dough with your fingertips. If the dough isn't quite reaching the edges of the pan, use your hands to stretch it.

5. Sprinkle the Italian seasoning and garlic over the top of the focaccia, and then place the pan in the center of your oven, allowing it to cook until golden, about twenty-five minutes. Remove the pans from the oven, and then use a spatula to remove the bread from the pan, transferring it to a wire cooling rack.

Cinnamon Swirl Loaf

This cinnamon swirl loaf is perfect on its own, but even better when it is used to make fresh toast in the mornings. You will love the fresh cinnamon flavor and find yourself making this delicious bread quite regularly.

Chronic Kidney Disease Stage: 1-5/Dialysis

The Details:

The Number of Servings: 4

The Time Needed to Prepare: 30 minutes

The Time Required to Cook: 30 minutes

The Total Preparation/Cook Time: 60 minutes

Number of Calories In Individual Servings: 326

Protein Grams: 7

Phosphorus Milligrams: 77

Potassium Milligrams: 87

Sodium Milligrams: 3

Fat Grams: 10

Total Carbohydrates Grams: 49

Net Carbohydrates Grams: 46

The Ingredients:

- All-purpose flour – 2 cups
- Water, warm - .75 cup
- Active dry yeast – 1.25 teaspoons

- Olive oil, light tasting – 3 tablespoons

- Cinnamon, ground – 1 tablespoon

- Truvia sweetener – 4 tablespoons

The Instructions:

1. Combine the warm water and active dry yeast together in a large bowl, whisking them until the yeast is dissolved. Allow this mixture to rest for five to ten minutes until the yeast is foam-like and bubbly.

2. Once the yeast has poofed, add in half of the Truvia, half of the olive oil, and the flour. Using the dough, hook on your stand mixer and combine this for three minutes. You will know that the dough is ready when it is soft yet pulls away from the sides of the bowl without sticking. If needed, you can add extra flour until it reaches this consistency.

3. Continue to knead the dough in the stand mixer until it is smooth and elastic, about seven minutes. Be careful to not over-knead the dough or it will turn tough.

4. Cover the bowl with plastic wrap and allow the dough to rise in a warm location until it has doubled in size, about thirty minutes.

5. Preheat your oven to a Fahrenheit temperature of three-hundred and fifty degrees and lightly grease a nine-by-five inch loaf pan. In a small bowl, combine the remaining half of the Truvia and the cinnamon.

6. Punch down the dough and then roll it into a rectangle nine inches long. Brush the dough with the remaining olive oil and then sprinkle the Truvia and cinnamon mixture over the dough.

7. Starting at the short side of the dough, begin to roll it into a tight log resembling cinnamon rolls.

8. Transfer the prepared cinnamon dough to the loaf pan, cover it with plastic wrap, and allow it to rise in a warm location for thirty minutes.

9. Place the risen dough in the preheated oven and allow it to bake until the dough is light and sounds hollow when tapped on about forty minutes. Remove the bread from the oven, let it rest for ten minutes, and then remove it from the pan, allowing it to cool on a wire cooling rack. Cool the bread completely before cutting it.

French Bread

Chronic Kidney Disease Stage: 1-5/Dialysis

The Details:

The Number of Servings: 6

The Time Needed to Prepare: 30 minutes

The Time Required to Cook: 30 minutes

The Total Preparation/Cook Time: 60 minutes

Number of Calories In Individual Servings: 330

Protein Grams: 8

Phosphorus Milligrams: 86

Potassium Milligrams: 98

Sodium Milligrams: 8

Fat Grams: 7

Total Carbohydrates Grams: 56

Net Carbohydrates Grams: 54

The Ingredients:

- All-purpose flour – 3.25 cups
- Warm water – .25 cup
- Hot water – 1 cup
- Active dry yeast – 1 tablespoon
- Honey – 1.5 tablespoons
- Olive oil – 3 tablespoons
- Egg white – 1 tablespoon

The Instructions:

1. In a large measuring cup, whisk the yeast and warm water together until it is dissolved. Be sure that the measuring cup isn't too small or else the liquid might expand too much and overflow. Allow the yeast to poof in the water for ten minutes, until it has expanded and become foam-like.

2. In a large bowl, mix together the hot water with the honey, olive oil, and half of the flour. Add in the yeast water that is done proofing. Slowly add in the remaining flour and continue to stir until the dough pulls away from the edges of the bowl. Allow the dough to sit for ten minutes.

3. On a floured surface, roll the dough into a long rectangle rolled up like a jelly roll and shaped like a French bread loaf. Smooth out the edges of the dough. Transfer the loaf onto a prepared greased baking sheet and use a knife to cut four diagonal on the bread.

4. Using a pastry brush, coat the loaf with the egg white, which will give it a nice golden color during the baking process.

5. Allow the bread loaf to sit in a warm location, not covered, for forty minutes until it has risen quite a bit. Then, place it in a preheated oven set to Fahrenheit three-hundred and seventy-five degrees until it is golden, cooked through, and sounds hollow when you knock on it, about twenty to twenty-five minutes.

6. Remove the bread from the oven and allow it to cool completely before slicing.

Chapter 9: Desserts

While desserts should always be enjoyed in moderation, the desserts in this chapter have been created to be ideal for the kidney disease diet. While most desserts are full of sugar, these use natural alternative sweeteners that won't negatively affect blood sugar, and it keeps saturated fats from butter to a minimum. This means that if your chronic kidney disease is caused by diabetes or high blood pressure, you can still enjoy these desserts.

Cinnamon Apple Crisp

This apple crisp is perfect for autumn or any other day of the year. You will absolutely love how easy it is to assemble and bake, allowing you to have an inexpensive and delicious dessert in only a few minutes.

Chronic Kidney Disease Stage: 1-5/Dialysis

The Details:

The Number of Servings: 2

The Time Needed to Prepare: 10 minutes

The Time Required to Cook: 25 minutes

The Total Preparation/Cook Time: 35 minutes

Number of Calories In Individual Servings: 496

Protein Grams: 9

Phosphorus Milligrams: 180

Potassium Milligrams: 269

Sodium Milligrams: 5

Fat Grams: 18

Total Carbohydrates Grams: 77

Net Carbohydrates Grams: 71

The Ingredients:

- Apples, peeled and sliced – 2 cups
- Lemon juice – 1 teaspoon
- Truvia sweetener - .25 cup
- Cinnamon - .5 teaspoon
- All-purpose flour – 1 cup, plus 2 tablespoons
- Rolled oats - .25 cup
- Brown sugar Truvia sweetener - .3 tablespoons
- Butter, cold, cut into pieces – 3 tablespoons

The Instructions:

1. Preheat your oven to a Fahrenheit temperature of three-hundred and fifty degrees Fahrenheit.

2. Lay out your sliced apples in a loaf pan and then toss them with the lemon juice, cinnamon, and the regular Truvia sweetener.

3. In a small bowl, combine the flour and cold butter with either a pastry cutter or a fork until it creates a crumbly mixture. Add in the brown

sugar Truvia and the oatmeal, and then sprinkle this crumble mixture over the apple slices.

4. Place the loaf pan in the oven and bake the crisp for twenty-five to thirty minutes, until the apples are tender and the topping is golden brown. Enjoy the crisp while it is still warm.

Vanilla Chia Seed Pudding

This pudding is quick and easy, but extremely delicious! Not only can it be made with strawberries, but other fruits as well! Customize this pudding to fit your taste or make it according to the recipe, either way, it is delicious.

Chronic Kidney Disease Stage: 1-5/Dialysis

The Details:

The Number of Servings: 2

The Time Needed to Prepare: 5 minutes

The Time Required to Cook: 0 minutes

The Total Preparation/Cook Time: 5 minutes

Number of Calories In Individual Servings: 106

Protein Grams: 3

Phosphorus Milligrams: 143

Potassium Milligrams: 135

Sodium Milligrams: 66

Fat Grams: 5

Total Carbohydrates Grams: 7

Net Carbohydrates Grams: 2

The Ingredients:

- Almond milk, vanilla, unsweetened - .75 cup
- Chia seeds – 4 tablespoons
- Vanilla extract – 2 teaspoons

- Truvia sweetener – 1 tablespoon

- Frozen strawberries, thawed – 3 ounces

The Instructions:

1. In a small jar, combine the chia seeds, unsweetened vanilla almond milk, vanilla extract, and Truvia sweetener. Ensure that the mixture is well combined so that the chia seeds don't form clumps. Allow this mixture to chill in the refrigerator for four to eight hours before enjoying. You might need to stir the mixture occasionally as it chills to ensure the chia seeds don't begin to stick together.

2. In a blender, puree the thawed strawberries, and then pour this puree over the chilled and set chia pudding. Enjoy the pudding immediately or store it in the fridge for up to four days.

Raspberry Frozen Yogurt

Whenever you are craving ice cream, all you have to do is reach for your blender to enjoy this raspberry frozen yogurt. Enjoy it either alone or with the addition of a little chocolate.

Chronic Kidney Disease Stage: 1-5/Dialysis

The Details:

The Number of Servings: 2

The Time Needed to Prepare: 5 minutes

The Time Required to Cook: 0 minutes

The Total Preparation/Cook Time: 5 minutes

Number of Calories In Individual Servings: 139

Protein Grams: 8

Phosphorus Milligrams: 123

Potassium Milligrams: 260

Sodium Milligrams: 27

Fat Grams: 0

Total Carbohydrates Grams: 27

Net Carbohydrates Grams: 22

The Ingredients:

- Raspberries, frozen – 6 ounces
- Greek yogurt, plain – .5 cup
- Lemon juice – 3 tablespoons

- Honey – 1.5 tablespoons

- Lemon zest – 1 teaspoon

The Instructions:

1. In a blender, combine the frozen raspberries, Greek yogurt, lemon juice, and honey until it forms a smooth and even consistency.

2. Either enjoy the frozen yogurt immediately for a soft-serve texture or place it in the freezer for one to two hours for a more solid consistency.

Skinny Cheesecake

This cheesecake is made much healthier by using a base of low-fat cream cheese and Greek yogurt, which is combined with Truvia as a sugar-free sweetener. This cheesecake is incredibly easy to make, and even someone new to the kitchen can follow this simple recipe.

Chronic Kidney Disease Stage: 1-5/Dialysis

The Details:

The Number of Servings: 6

The Time Needed to Prepare: 10 minutes

The Time Required to Cook: 60 minutes

The Total Preparation/Cook Time: 70 minutes

Number of Calories In Individual Servings: 199

Protein Grams: 8

Phosphorus Milligrams: 135

Potassium Milligrams: 182

Sodium Milligrams: 195

Fat Grams: 13

Total Carbohydrates Grams: 10

Net Carbohydrates Grams: 10

The Ingredients:

- Cream cheese, low-fat, at room temperature – 8 ounces

- Greek yogurt, fat-free – 1 cup

- Egg – 1
- Truvia sweetener - .33 cup
- Vanilla extract – 1 teaspoon
- Graham crackers – 1.5 ounces
- Olive oil, light tasting – 3 tablespoons

The Instructions:

1. Preheat your oven to a Fahrenheit temperature of three-hundred and fifty degrees and grease a five-inch round baking pan.

2. Place your graham crackers into a food processor and pulse them until they reach a uniform and fine crumb. Add in the light olive oil and pulse again until the fat is combined into the crumbs. Pour the crumb mixture into the prepared baking pan and firmly press down the cookie crumbs into the pan to form a crust. Set the pan aside while you make the cheesecake filling.

3. Clean the food processor, and then pulse together the Greek yogurt, cream cheese, Truvia, and vanilla extract. Process this mixture until it is fully combined, about one minute.

4. Add the egg into the food processor and pulse for a few seconds more to fully incorporate it into the cream cheese and yogurt base. Be careful not to over mix the cheesecake, as that will cause the top to crack during the cooking process.

5. Pour the cheesecake batter into the prepared graham cracker crust and allow it to cook in the preheated oven for thirty minutes. After the thirty minutes is up turn the oven off, leave the oven door closed, and allow the cheesecake to sit in the hot oven that has been turned off for thirty additional minutes.

6. After the thirty minutes of sitting in the oven that is turned off, remove the cheesecake from the oven, and allow it to sit on the kitchen counter until it reaches room temperature, at least four hours. Once room temperature, cover the cheesecake with plastic wrap and allow it to chill in the refrigerator for eight hours before slicing and serving.

Lemon and Honey Oatmeal Cookies

These cookies taste fresh and bright from the honey and lemon, but with a wonderful depth from the oatmeal. You can either buy oat flour pre-made at the store, or you can make your own by simply running some oats through the food processor. Either way, you will find that these cookies are incredibly simple and quick to make.

Chronic Kidney Disease Stage: 1-5/Dialysis

The Details:

The Number of Servings: 3

The Time Needed to Prepare: 5 minutes

The Time Required to Cook: 12 minutes

The Total Preparation/Cook Time: 17 minutes

Number of Calories In Individual Servings: 262

Protein Grams: 7

Phosphorus Milligrams: 297

Potassium Milligrams: 311

Sodium Milligrams: 15

Fat Grams: 8

Total Carbohydrates Grams: 41

Net Carbohydrates Grams: 38

The Ingredients:

- Quick oats - .5 cup
- Oat flour – 6 tablespoons

- Baking powder, low sodium - .75 teaspoon
- Coconut oil – 1 tablespoon
- Honey – 2.5 tablespoons
- Vanilla extract – 1 teaspoon
- Lemon juice – 1 teaspoon
- Lemon zest - .25 teaspoon
- Liquid egg – 1.5 tablespoons

The Instructions:

1. In a medium bowl, combine the quick oats, low-sodium baking powder, and the oat flour.

2. In another bowl, whisk together the liquid egg, honey, coconut oil, lemon zest, vanilla extract, and lemon juice.

3. Add the wet ingredients to the dry and combine the two until they are fully incorporated. Cover the bowl with plastic wrap or a lid and allow it to chill in the refrigerator for thirty minutes.

4. Preheat your oven to a Fahrenheit temperature of three-hundred and twenty-five degrees and line a baking sheet with kitchen parchment.

5. Using a spoon, create six evenly-sized mounds of dough on the prepared baking sheet, each round of dough being one to two inches apart so that the cookies don't meld into each other. Use a fork and flatten the dough out into disks.

6. Bake the cookies in your preheated oven for twelve minutes, until they are set and starting

to turn golden. Be careful to not overcook them. Remove the pan from the oven and carefully transfer the cookies to a wire rack to cool. Enjoy while warm or store them for later.

Carrot Cake Cookies

These carrot cake cookies are free of oils and granulated sugar, instead of using a small amount of honey and unsweetened apple sauce. Whether you are wanting these as a special dessert or a snack to take on-the-go, any fan of carrot cake will love these cookies!

Chronic Kidney Disease Stage: 1-5/Dialysis

The Details:

The Number of Servings: 3

The Time Needed to Prepare: 5 minutes

The Time Required to Cook: 12 minutes

The Total Preparation/Cook Time: 17 minutes

Number of Calories In Individual Servings: 179

Protein Grams: 5

Phosphorus Milligrams: 159

Potassium Milligrams: 187

Sodium Milligrams: 9

Fat Grams: 5

Total Carbohydrates Grams: 29

Net Carbohydrates Grams: 26

The Ingredients:

- Carrot, peeled and sliced – 1
- Honey – 3 tablespoons
- Apple sauce, unsweetened - .5 cup
- Rolled oats – 1 cup

- Walnuts, chopped - .25 cup
- Cinnamon, ground .5 teaspoon
- Ginger, ground - .5 teaspoon
- Nutmeg, ground - .25 teaspoon

The Instructions:

1. Preheat your oven to a Fahrenheit temperature of three-hundred and seventy-five degrees and line a baking sheet with kitchen parchment.

2. In a food processor, blend the carrots until they form a fine meal. Add in the honey, apple sauce, rolled oats, walnuts, cinnamon, ginger, and nutmeg. With the food processor, do five quick pulses, being careful to avoid over blending the mixture. Remove the blade from the food processor and use a spatula to finish combining the mixture.

3. Use a spoon or a small cookie scoop to make your cookie dough balls, each one containing two tablespoons of cookie dough. Use your hands to form the dough into two-inch disks and place these disks a couple of inches apart on the prepared baking sheet.

4. Place your baking sheet in the oven and allow the cookies to cook until they form a deep golden color around the edges, about twenty-five to thirty minutes.

5. Remove the pan from the oven and allow them to cool for five minutes before transferring the cookies to a wire cooling rack to complete the cooling process.

Conclusion

You likely had little knowledge about your kidneys before. You probably didn't know how you could take steps to improve your kidney health and decrease the risk of developing kidney failure. However, through reading this book, you now understand the power of the human kidney, as well as the prognosis of chronic kidney disease. While over thirty-million Americans are being affected by kidney disease, you can now take steps to be one of the people who is actively working to promote your kidney health.

With the help of Dr. Robert Porter and Dr. Elizabeth Torres, you now have all the information you need to succeed. You understand your kidney health better, you have learned of some of the new therapies now available and in the research stages, and you have been given over sixty recipes that can help you attain success and better health. Not only can these recipes help you improve your kidney functioning, decrease the risk of kidney disease, decrease mortality risk, and treat common conditions that coincide with kidney disease, but these recipes also taste amazing and can be incorporated into any healthy lifestyle.

If you found the knowledge and information imparted by Dr. Porter and the delicious and nutritious recipes shared by Dr. Torres helpful, then you should check out their other book. Their book**, _Kidney Disease Diet,_** will give you even more information on the biological function of kidneys, how chronic kidney disease and other kidney diseases affect your health, the prognosis of chronic kidney disease, and how you can take further steps, both with your diet and lifestyle, to better your health.

Thank you for reading the *Renal Diet Cookbook*. We hope that with the information you have learned, you will soon gain a healthier and happier lifestyle. You can enjoy gaining healthier kidneys, lower blood pressure, reduced cholesterol, and healthier blood sugar. By combining this book and a doctor's consultation, you can live better and longer.

Made in the USA
Columbia, SC
10 May 2020

96076762R00186